Growth in Childhood

T0321439

Growth in Childhood

Edited by

Terence J. Wilkin

Reader in Endocrinology, Department of Medicine II,
University of Southampton, UK

A collection of essays based on a series of lectures
given at a symposium held at the University of
Southampton Medical School.

harwood academic publishers
chur · london · paris · new york · melbourne

Harwood Academic Publishers

Post Office Box 197
London WC2E 9PX
England

58, rue Lhomond
75005 Paris
France

Post Office Box 786
Cooper Station
New York, New York 10276
United States of America

Private Bag 8
Camberwell, Victoria 3124
Australia

Library of Congress Cataloging-in-Publication Data

Growth in childhood.

Bibliography: p.
Includes index.
1. Children—Growth.   2. Growth disorders—Treatment.
I. Wilkin, Terence J.
RJ131.G77   1989   618.92   89–15223′
ISBN 3–7186–4941–1

Contents

Preface

With the description in 1985 of three fatalities due to Jakob–Creutzfeldt disease caused by slow virus infection of human pituitary growth hormone preparations, the need for recombinant growth hormone became acute. The marketing of synthetic growth hormone later that year heralded a new era in the treatment of growth failure since growth hormone although expensive, was now available in limitless quantities. The restrictions in application which characterised the era of cadaveric growth hormone evaporated. A new interest and new energy in the investigation of growth deficiency has emerged, with a new literature in the therapeutic implications of growth hormone treatment. This involves not only growth hormone deficiency, growth failure associated with Turner's syndrome and achondroplasia but many other circumstances which were previously beyond the reach of growth hormone treatment. The reports of new applications for growth hormone therapy have been accompanied by renewed awareness in the physiology of growth and understanding of growth factors.

There are many excellent texts concerned with the problems of growth in childhood, but this does not aim to be a textbook. Drawing on the edited transcripts from a symposium on "Growth in Childhood" this is a series of essays that covers a wide range of topics in a concise, chatty form. This book is not aimed at specialists in growth but at those with an interest in endocrinology and pediatrics who wish to extend their general knowledge of the subject. Beginning with an introduction concerned with the measurement of growth, the book deals with areas of growth management which should appeal as much to medical students as to general practitioners and hospital clinicians.

T. J. Wilkin

Contributors

Professor G. Michael Besser
Professor of Endocrinology, The Medical College of
St. Bartholomew's Hospital, West Smithfield, London, UK

Dr Peter R. Betts
Consultant Paediatrician, Level G, East Wing, Southampton
General Hospital, Southampton, UK

Dr Charles G. D. Brook
Reader in Paediatric Endocrinology, Cobbold Laboratories,
The Middlesex Hospital, Mortimer Street, London, UK

Dr John M. H. Buckler
Senior Lecturer in Paediatrics and Consultant Paediatrician,
University Department of Paediatrics and Child Health,
D Floor, Clarendon Wing, The General Infirmary at Leeds,
Belmont Grove, Leeds, UK

Mr Tam Fry
Honorary Chairman, Child Growth Foundation,
2 Mayfield Avenue, Chiswick, London, UK

Dr Brian A. Gennery
Lilly Research Centre Ltd, Group Medical Director (Europe),
Earl Wood Manor, Windlesham, Surrey, UK

Dr J. Michael Parkin
Reader in Paediatrics
Department of Child Health,
The Medical School, Framlington Place,
Newcastle upon Tyne, UK

Dr Richard Ross
The Medical College of St. Bartholomew's Hospital,
West Smithfield, London, UK

Dr Martin O. Savage
Consultant Paediatric Endocrinologist,
Department of Child Health,
St. Bartholomew's Hospital, West Smithfield,
London, UK

Dr Stephen Wise
Lilly Research Centre Ltd,
Erl Wood Manor,
Windlesham, Surrey, UK

Growth Measurement

JOHN BUCKLER

Senior Lecturer in Paediatrics and Consultant Paediatrician, University Department of Paediatrics and Child Health, D Floor, Clarendon Wing, The General Infirmary at Leeds, Belmont Grove, Leeds LS2 9NS, UK

A review is presented of the history of growth measurements and surveys of growth. The relevance of growth measurements, the importance of accuracy in longitudinal observations and the factors associated with accuracy are discussed. The use of centile charts and what determines their appropriateness are considered.

KEY WORDS: Anthropometry, auxology, puberty, growth spurt, growth studies, accuracy, centiles

HISTORICAL BACKGROUND

In discussing the subject of the history of growth measurement, reference must be made to the writings of Professor Tanner, to whom I am indebted not only for my personal interest in and knowledge of auxology but, in this particular context, for his excellent book "A History of the Study of Human Growth" (Cambridge University Press, 1981), a comprehensive and invaluable source of material upon which I have drawn extensively. This volume provides the interested reader with as much information as he could possibly want.

Prior to the last 200 years or so, interest in the physical body and its growth was related much more to body proportions than to actual size. Elsholtz, a German physician, in the mid 1600's first used the term anthropometry and devised an anthropometer whose mechanism was much more orientated to demonstrating relative size of components of body height than the actual height itself. It was not until 1795 with the introduction of the metre that there was any precise length standard, and values for length had no consistent basis and varied from place to place.

The importance of height for military recruits in the 18th and 19th centuries was a reason for the development of interest in height as such,

1

and Goethe, at one stage being involved in recruiting, drew a sketch in 1779 demonstrating remarkably good measuring technique.

The first and still one of the best recorded longitudinal studies of growth, now very familiar, was the record by Count Montbeillard of the growth of his son in the years 1759–77, made at the request of Buffon and published in the 4th set of 7 volumes of his supplements to the Natural History. There is no comment on the measurement techniques except that all were undertaken by Montbeillard himself at 6-monthly intervals and with his son barefoot, and the graphical presentation and derived height velocities indicate the precision and care of his methods.

The Belgian genius Quetelet, whose interests covered a vast range of scientific subjects and who undertook the first population survey of children in 1831–32, also recorded the longitudinal growth data of two of his own children and two daughters of friends. He would not, however, recognize the apparent growth spurt, but smoothed his curves, being convinced that "l'homme moyen (average man), at least, should have a growth curve of perfect regularity and impeccable form." (Tanner).

Others through the years have measured their own children and one of the most meticulous was Christian Wiener (who used the concept of decimal age 100 years before Tanner) who measured his 4 sons between 1856–90, initially annually, but with greater enthusiasm and frequency as new ones appeared, so that the last was measured 89 times. These sons showed unequivocal growth spurts, but interesting variations in the ages of peak height velocity, 13.2, 13.5, 14.5 and 12.5 years.

[A rather more recent family study is now presented of my own three boys measured through the years of puberty, which shows a similar variation, with peaks at 13.5, 14.2 and 15.2 years, Figures 1–3.]

In England epidemiological growth studies were first carried out as the result of the Factory Commission of 1833. These studies measured the heights of 2000 boys and girls who had worked in a factory from an early age, and demonstrated that these children were stunted. Subsequently Charles Roberts took an interest in the growth of children through his involvement in a Parliamentary Commission in 1872–73 studying the growth and welfare of nearly 10 000 North of England factory and other working class children. He demonstrated a striking difference between the heights of the children of manual and non-

BOYS HEIGHT

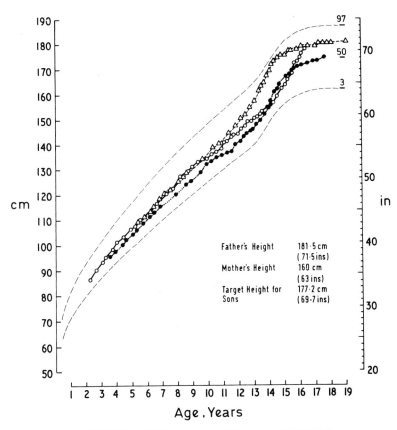

FIGURE 1   Height centiles of 3 brothers (1974–1987).

manual workers. Roberts also observed the great variation around the mean, and noted how misleading mere averages could be.

Francis Galton, about the same time as Roberts, transformed the study of growth in this country. Recognizing the need for information countrywide about children's growth he sponsored in 1873 a programme of body measurements in schools. He developed a stadiometer basically the same as the modern Harpenden instrument and interpreted distribution in these accurately obtained values in terms corresponding

BOYS WEIGHT

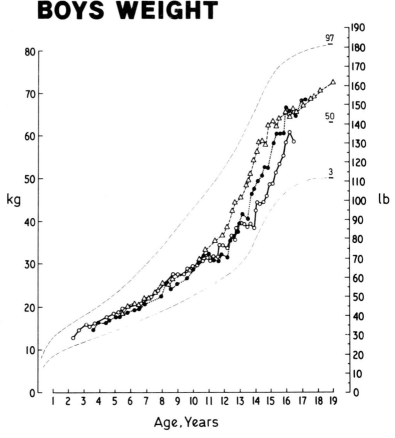

FIGURE 2   Weight centiles of 3 brothers.

to standard deviation. He also developed other important statistical concepts. Through a large family study of nearly 10 000 persons he was able to demonstrate the importance of familial factors in growth, and showed how to present data in terms of centiles. He also interpreted, years before anyone else, the misleading effects in growth curves at puberty of averaging cross-sectional data, and stressed the need for longitudinal growth studies on individuals.

In the USA interest in growth started with the work of Henry Bowditch, who in 1872 presented 25 years worth of growth data of 25

BOYS HEIGHT VELOCITY

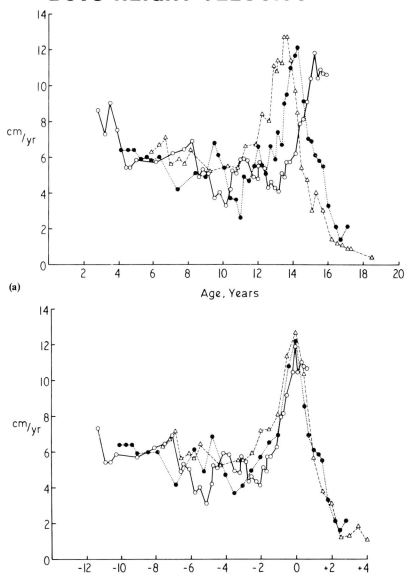

(a)

(b)

FIGURE 3 Height velocity centiles of 3 brothers. (a) Plotted according to chronological age. (b) Plotted in relation to the ages of peak height velocity.

closely related individuals. He went on to undertake a massive survey in state and private schools (24 500 children) and presented data as height charts through the years. He noted the different timing of the growth of boys and girls but, like many others, he missed the significance of the different growth patterns of early and late developers in explaining differences between social or ethnic groups.

[Bowditch's studies were followed up in other areas of the States by Peckham and Porter, the latter pointing out (1920) that centiles represented what the overall distribution was, not what it necessarily should be.]

Schools surveys had also been undertaken in other countries, notably by Pagliani in Italy who in a paper in 1897 demonstrated the growth spurt following the period of slowest growth, but he was the first to recognize the significance of the different timing of pubertal growth in individuals, which effect is obscured in composite means. He showed, contrary to his predecessors, that puberty (reproduction) and growth go in parallel, both dependent on the same underlying influence, as illustrated in girls by the growth spurt being linked in time with menarche, preceding it by between 1 and 2 years, whatever the age of menarche. Following Pagliani, school surveys were undertaken in many other parts of Europe and by 1900 growth curves were available for many countries.

The credit for first recognition of the significance of the difference between individual and composite growth patterns is however usually given to Frank Boas who as well as initiating the first large longitudinal growth study also produced in 1898 composite North American standards based on about 90 000 children. However in 1892, shortly after Pagliani and independently, he pointed out that almost all individuals deviate from the composite centile position at puberty, but not until 1930 did he show that each individual has a maximum growth age, demonstrated by velocity curves which vary over a wide age range among the population of adolescents. It was he, probably, who originated the term "physiological age". He showed that early developing boys were taller by age 11, but did not necessarily end up taller, and the earlier the age of maximum growth rate, the higher was this peak height velocity.

Boas' work was confirmed and followed up very soon by the massive Harvard longitudinal growth study, started in 1923, in which nearly 1000 children were measured annually from age 6 to 18. This was reported by Frank Shuttleworth in 1937 in a very comprehensive monograph which forms the basis of the modern understanding and appreciation of growth studies. He emphasized the need for the vast potential information of longitudinal studies to be used to demonstrate increments of growth, i.e. velocities, rather than losing this information in cross sectional presentation of gross measurements. He showed the value of comparing individuals' velocity curves for each parameter in terms of maximum growth age. This enabled demonstration of relationships of timing of growth of different body dimensions, and comparison of growth patterns of early and late developers. Surprisingly Shuttleworth's writings did not correlate growth patterns with secondary sexual characteristics, which had first been used in a graded way by the pioneer in growth surveillance, the French physician Paul Godin, in the early years of this century.

The importance of rating and relating secondary sexual characteristics has been much emphasized in the more recent Harpenden Growth study of Tanner and Whitehouse. This is a very comprehensive study undertaken on 228 boys and 192 girls between the years 1948 and 1971, with frequent observations through the years of puberty. In addition to presentation of growth data of many other body dimensions than just height and weight, interrelationships are demonstrated and in particular the range of variation of pubic hair, genital and breast development, graded according to the widely used descriptions of Tanner. The accuracy of measurements is established by the fact that they were all undertaken throughout by one observer only, Whitehouse himself, using instruments which he had personally designed and whose accuracy far surpassed those previously in use whose design had been unchanged for many decades.

THE NEED FOR GROWTH MEASUREMENT

Only by measurement is it possible to recognize the significance of dimensions of individuals and groups when these are compared appropriately against standards of overall populations. Mere impressions can be very misleading. Bowditch in 1881 pointed out that there was value in measurement in two directions, in the comparative health of populations and large scale identification of deprived areas and also in the recognition of growth problems of individuals. During this century numerous school surveys have been carried out in the Western world and such large scale surveys have established many general fundamental facts such as the adverse effects of overcrowding. It is important, however, to stress the distinction between comparisons of populations which indicate the need for improvements in general social and health standards, and observations on individuals which indicate the need for specific treatment.

Some countries have pioneered in population growth monitoring, notably several surveys in Holland since 1955. Little was done in Britain prior to 1972, but since that time, as the result of concern emanating from the restriction of free milk in schools, the National Study of Health and Growth has monitored growth in primary school children aged 5–11 and the Pre-School Child Growth Survey in children from birth to 5 years. These surveys are still continuing.

One of the pioneers in recognizing the value of measurement in both these aspects, the relevance to the group and to the individual, was Paul Godin who in 1919 first coined the term "auxology" which he defined as "the study of growth by the method of following the same subjects during numerous six-monthly periods with a great number of measurements". Godin's meticulous application of measurements has, as Tanner points out, only been equalled by Whitehouse. Godin personally undertook 129 measurements on each boy on about 1000 total boy–occasions (very similar to Whitehouse's total of 15 measurements on 9000 child–occasions). Single measurements correctly interpreted on centile charts may well be the trigger that alerts an observer to a potential problem, but serial measurements that show a fall off in growth velocity are of greater value and provide one of the surest signs of ill health.

THE DIFFICULTIES IN OBTAINING RELIABLE SERIAL MEASUREMENTS

The need for accuracy

A relatively minor degree of inaccuracy in any measurement in the "one-off" observation circumstance may not be critical or render the observation valueless. The effect of this degree of error when plotted to give a centile position may be relatively trivial, and is unlikely to be so great as to alter the interpretation of its significance or to miss recognizing the need for concern and action. Recording such values for reference in the distant future will also provide useful information (particularly if the limitations of the technique are recognized), for if the interval between observations is long enough, the effect of inaccuracy will be small compared with the overall expected growth change, and deviation from centile positions would still be apparent..

However, in those situations where these initial measurements have given rise for concern, the need for frequent follow-up becomes highly important and with it the need for as great a degree of accuracy as possible. An error which is lost in the overall accumulated growth of several years is highly significant over intervals of a few months or even a year and inaccurate measurements may cause totally erroneous conclusions to be drawn about growth patterns in terms of parallelism to centile lines or lack of it.

Height or length should not ever have negative velocities through the growing years (with certain provisos mentioned subsequently), whereas weight is often lost over short periods without necessarily implying ill health, and interpretation of such short term changes requires a somewhat different approach.

FACTORS RELEVANT IN THE ACCURACY AND VALUE OF MEASUREMENTS

Many variations in measurements are avoidable, some are not, but the observer needs to be aware of them and where possible take them into account.

Equipment

A measurement can only be as accurate as the equipment allows. Systems for measuring height or length only to the nearest half or completed centimetre cannot be used to evaluate small changes. In addition, instruments need to be checked regularly against standards to ensure that the given values remain correct.

Technique

The correct methods of measurement are those described by Tanner, and substantial error will occur if the techniques are not applied. Fundamentally height measurement requires the subject to be barefoot, standing vertical against a firm upright, as tall as possible but with the feet flat on the ground so that the heels are not raised, without any tilt of the head or shrugging of the shoulders, and stretched with gentle traction by upward pressure under the ears.

Inter- and intra-observer variation

Repeated measurements by the same experienced measurer should be very similar, differences in height usually not exceeding 3 mm. This is a highly reproducible measurement, but differences in other linear measurements are unavoidably greater. However, the difference between measurers, even the most experienced, may be considerable, perhaps mostly dependent on how "gentle upward traction" is interpreted. It is no secret that even in the most prestigious centre of anthropometry differences of half a centimetre or even more in height may be found between the height measurements of the "experts". With tall subjects, measurement of height and the application of appropriate upward traction becomes more difficult, particularly if the measurer is not very tall himself.

These observations show how much more reliable are measurements undertaken by the same observer on each occasion, for his technique should be consistent. This applies not only to large-scale longitudinal growth studies such as those of Godin and Whitehouse, but also to clinical situations in the evaluation of the growth of an individual, though in practice this ideal may not always be easy to achieve.

Time of day

That individuals shrink as the day proceeds is a fact that has been known for many years, though not widely recognized. Reverend Joseph Wasse, an English vicar, in 1724 discoursed very fully on the loss of height amounting to an inch through the course of the day, which he attributed to the "yielding of the cartilage between the vertebrae". In

Montbeillard's famous report of the growth of his own son (1749) (as quoted by Tanner), he noted an apparent decrease of height when measured the morning after an all-night dance, a decrease that disappeared by the following morning. Christian Wiener in the longitudinal study of his own son reported in 1890 also demonstrated a reduction in height of 4 to 7 mm during the day.

This reduction of height is mainly in the spine, and the purpose of upward traction on the head in modern height measurement techniques is to compensate for this shrinkage that happens throughout the day, but this it does not fully do. In a simple study of my own I measured, by the standard technique with neck traction, about 10 schoolboys at intervals throughout 24 hours, and showed a reduction in height in them all. All were tallest on getting out of bed in the morning and within an hour height had fallen by about 1 cm. Throughout the day there was a gradual continuing decrement of about a further cm, the shortest height being not surprisingly on retiring to bed at night. By the following morning the full 2 cm was always regained.

This observation has considerable implications, though it is not always possible to avoid the problem. Clearly it is inadvisable to use in serial observations height measurements taken on first rising from bed (which could happen in a hospital setting) and ideally in the clinical situation, subjects should be seen on regular visits at about the same time of day. This is not always practical, but unexpected changes in height velocity could sometimes be accounted for by a different time of observation through the day.

One important aspect is that there comes an age in any young growing child when he becomes cooperative enough for measurement of length to be changed to height. That will result in a reduction of the measurement by about 1 cm, and on the standard Tanner growth charts this change is shown at the age of 2 years, but in practice this precise age may not always be the most appropriate. It is clearly important, however, to note in serial records on a centile chart at what age this actual change occurs to avoid misinterpretation of height changes.

Season of the year

It has been recognized that growth rates in many children vary according to the time of year, being faster in spring and summer than in autumn and winter. This is easier to document in prepubertal children than in those whose height velocity is rapidly changing during the course of puberty. This was yet another observation that Montbeillard was probably the first to make on the growth of his son, and it was reported by Buffon that total growth in the age period 5–10 years was 19.2 cm in the summer months and only 11.2 cm in the winter ones.

In the 1880's the Danish worker, Malling-Hansen, over a period of two years measured daily at 9.00 a.m. the weights and heights of about 70 boys aged 9–15 and showed a maximum growth rate in spring time (5.6 mm/month) that was two-and-a-half times greater than the minimum rate in the autumn (2.3 mm/month). Weight changes were in the opposite direction, maximum being in the autumn and minimum in the spring. These findings have been confirmed many times since and the modern values reported by Marshall from Tanner's department in 1971 were very similar to those of Montbeillard.

Frequency of observations

The average boy or girl in the years preceding puberty increases height by only 5–6 cm per year on average, less than 5 mm per month (though varying through the course of the year). It is therefore apparent that with all these factors which may influence a height measurement, many unavoidably, there is little value in measurement of height more frequent than 3-monthly, and in many situations where delay is not critical, comparison of heights over a full year will be most meaningful, thus avoiding error due to seasonal change. In many longitudinal studies, though measurements may be taken as frequently as every 3 or 4 months, velocities are calculated on the basis of the difference between those measurements a year apart.

PROBLEMS WITH ATTENDANCE AND COOPERATION

Serial observations on growing children, whether in the individual clinical follow-up or the large numbered group study, are fraught with difficulties in attendance through lack of interest, motivation, moving home or school, or sheer practicality. In longitudinal studies, whenever involvement is voluntary, subjects inevitably are lost and greatest successes are achieved where the group is to some extent "captive" in a residential setting.

There is a great need for the monitoring of growth of as many children as possible within a country or area, not only to identify early those individuals with growth problems but also to ensure that adequate information can be acquired to prepare standards of growth appropriate to that overall population. Such widespread observations are not undertaken serially at present in this country, though they are in certain continental countries such as Germany, Austria and France, with personally held records. The success of this French "carnet" system is increased by financial inducement, for without cooperation mothers cannot obtain child benefit. In Britain, difficulties with recall and continued attendance related to the aims of prevention or early recognition of health problems are considerable and there is no consistent nationwide policy.

METHODS OF OBTAINING MEANINGFUL MEASUREMENTS

The facilities and equipment for measurement in schools and clinics throughout Britain vary greatly, but some degree of compromise must be accepted between what is optimal and what is practical. Every effort should be made to provide at low cost the means of assessing height and weight that are sufficiently reliable to allow comparable serial measurements to be interpreted correctly. This requires not only suitable equipment and knowledge of measurement technique, but also competent recording (with records that can be retrieved and referred to subsequently), appropriate centile charts in order to interpret the data and an understanding that will result in action and referral when appropriate.

In most situations measuring instruments or charts will need to be in a fixed position, as it is seldom practical or reliable to move measuring equipment from place to place. Fixed reliable height measuring equipment as found in hospital growth clinics (the Harpenden stadiometer) is too expensive for routine use elsewhere, and the introduction of various types of wall chart, e.g. Oxford Growth Screening Charts,

"See how I grow" (Marmite), has provided cheap, convenient alternatives for immediate identification of those whose height is outside the "average normal" range of the population, e.g. the 3rd or 97th centiles. These charts, which are essentially charts with height centiles plotted against age, require careful positioning at the correct height on the wall, which is not always easy, but then merely involves the child standing in front, without shoes, at the site of his particular age, so that his height centile is apparent. Though these charts provide immediate information on the significance of a height in terms of its centile, and so avoid the need for referring to centile charts elsewhere in order to interpret a height measurement, they are not ideal for providing the actual height recordings which form the basis of serial measurement.

The commonest wall-fixed height measuring apparatus are tape measures or a graduated vertical wooden upright to which a sliding horizontal head piece is fixed. Although in principle this latter is the basis of the stadiometer or anthropometer, in practice the headstick is liable to wobble over a considerable range and not slide smoothly on the upright, so that the alternative of resting a book held as horizontal as possible on the child's head and reading against a vertical tape or scale may be as reliable, or more so. The recent introduction of the "microtoise" has many advantages in its convenience, cheapness and relative accuracy, but again requires care in the placing of the hook from which it is suspended at exactly 2 metres from the floor.

In all these methods, other than the centile wall charts, the height as such means little until it is interpreted correctly on a centile chart. The limitations of a method in terms of accuracy must be recognized if follow-up measurements are envisaged, as the accuracy of these must be reasonable and the time interval between measurements sufficiently long if growth rates are to be interpreted correctly. Yet to do a height or length measurement at all in many settings is still quite an achievement. At a recent meeting attended by enthusiastic General Practitioners, less than a third undertook height measurements on children attending their surgeries.

THE USE OF APPROPRIATE CENTILE CHARTS

The fundamental for the interpretation of a child's growth pattern is the availability of correct standards of reference, and there may not be ideal centile charts for that particular child.

WHAT DETERMINES THE APPROPRIATENESS OF A CENTILE CHART?

Racial differences

Eveleth and Tanner have reported in great detail in their book "Worldwide Variation in Human Growth" (Cambridge University Press, 1976) the considerable racial differences in growth patterns and the influence on the growth of ethnic groups when they move to different parts of the world. It is inappropriate, though often unavoidable, to evaluate the growth of immigrant groups on the basis of the standards of the indigenous population.

Secular trends

As decades and centuries pass, so the growth of children changes, both within a country and world wide. The changes are manifest not only in differences in weight and height at any particular chronological age during the growing years, but also in the timing of puberty and its associated growth spurt, and in the ultimate sizes of adults. Many factors must be involved in these changes, some obvious, such as nutrition, socio-economic circumstances, wars, but others are less well defined.

Evidence from the earliest growth studies suggests that secular trends have occurred through the centuries, though they may occur both ways. In historical times of deprivation and misery, such as wars and the Dutch famine (1820–60), there was delay in growth and shortening of stature. Much of the apparent increase in size of children of comparable ages and sexes through the years is dependent on earlier puberty and the spurt of growth. This is illustrated by the age of menarche which, over the last century and until recently, has been advancing in most European countries, and in some Scandinavian countries as fast as 0.3 years per decade, or a year per generation. In the mid-nineteenth

JOHN BUCKLER

century menarche occurred on average at about 15 years in England
and 17 years in Scandinavia, whereas present European populations
show little variation between ages of menarche, mostly being about 13
years.

Middle class schoolboys in Britain of the same chronological age
became taller by about 1.5 cm per 10 years between 1880 and 1930
(and girls to a lesser extent), but the difference in adult height was far
less marked, indicating that the effect was primarily accounted for by
earlier maturing. These observations have also been made in other
European countries. Recent trends do not appear to be so dramatic,
but still exist. The British surveys since 1972 have shown an increase
in height of 0.77 cm per decade in English boys and 0.46 cm in English
girls, and 1.55 cm in Scottish boys and 0.58 cm in Scottish girls.

It is interesting to compare the standard 1959 Tanner charts with
the more recent ones of 1975 (Figures 4–5). Although the former are
plotted on the basis of cross sectional and the latter longitudinal
standards, it is clear there are considerable differences in height and
even more so in weight at comparable ages. The dramatic weight
changes in comparison to height might suggest that centiles, though
showing how a population distribution actually is, do not necessarily
represent what is optimal.

Socioeconomic differences

All reports through the centuries demonstrate that poverty and poorer
social circumstances are associated with shorter stature (weight being
less affected) and later maturation. One of the earliest records is of
pupils in the Carlschule in Stuttgart from 1772 to 1774. Despite similar
environment and nutrition at the school, the sons of nobility were
2.5 cm taller than the bourgeois at 10–11, 7 cm taller at 15, but only
1 cm taller at 20, indicating these differences were almost entirely due
to age of puberty.

Bowditch in the USA in his report in 1879, showed that "nonmanual"
boys were taller than "manual" by about 1-cm at 8–10, 2 cm at 11–12,
3 cm at 13–14 and 1 cm at 18, again clearly showing the effect of
difference in age of pubertal growth. The effect in girls was far less
marked, nonmanual being 1 cm taller at 13 than manual, but ending
up the same.

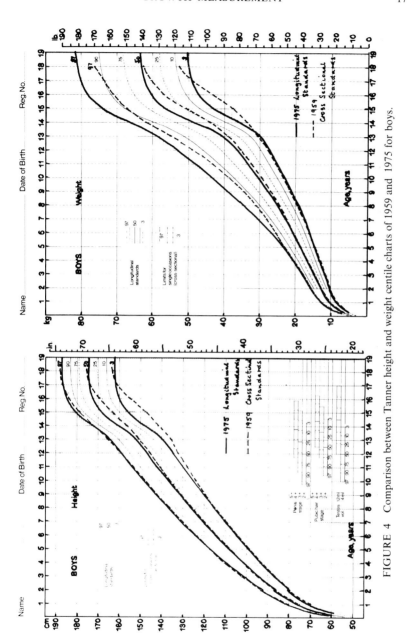

FIGURE 4   Comparison between Tanner height and weight centile charts of 1959 and 1975 for boys.

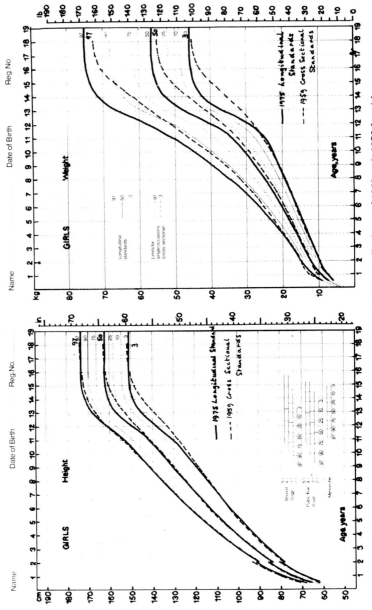

FIGURE 5   Comparison between Tanner height and weight centile charts of 1959 and 1975 for girls.

Roberts in England made very similar observations (1874–76) showing the difference between the boys of manual and nonmanual workers was about 6 cm at ages 9–11, 7 cm at 12, 9 cm at 13–14, 11 cm at 15–16, but only 5–6 cm at the final adult height, which was about 5 cm shorter than the average for similar social class nowadays. The age of maximal growth of the nonmanual group was 15.0 years compared with 16.0 in the manual group. The British studies in the 1970's suggest differences nowadays of 3 cm at ages 6–7, 4 cm at 11, and dropping to 3–3.5 cm at adult height, but the differences are greater in the subgroup who are particularly short (i.e. 3rd centile). Similar differences were found between the heights of children of fathers who were unemployed, who were on average 3.3 cm shorter than those of employed fathers of the same occupational class.

Geographical differences within a country

Heights and weights differ within the same racial groups in different regions of a country. In the 1965 Dutch survey, children in the North of the country were 3–4 cm taller than those in the South. Similar variations are found in Britain. A recent report on heights and weights of adults in Britain (1980) as well as showing the social class trends, showed greatest heights in the South of the country (except London GLC), the men averaging about 1.5 cm taller than in the North of the country and Scotland, and 3 cm taller than those in Wales. For women the comparable figures were 1.5 cm and 2.5 cm. It is probable that these values reflect similar differences during the growing years.

Whatever the cause for differences within a country, whether ethnic, social or geographical, there is a need for many further studies, and in particular a means of collating the information and disseminating it. I have recently reported the outcome of an analysis of the heights and weights of all Leeds children on whom data were available at school entry (around 5 years), and these measurements were comparable to those of Tanner (1965). However, it is interesting to read of growth surveys on 5-year-olds in Southampton and $3\frac{1}{2}$- to 10-year-olds in Edinburgh suggesting that they are considerably taller than Tanner's children of 20 years ago. There are plans for further surveys of schoolchildren in and around Leeds to provide a better picture of the differences in growth characteristics of ethnic minority groups.

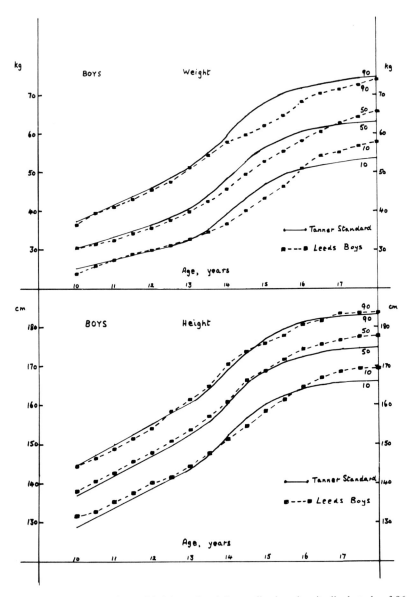

FIGURE 6 Comparison of height and weight centiles in a longitudinal study of 96 Leeds boys and Tanner's 1975 centiles.

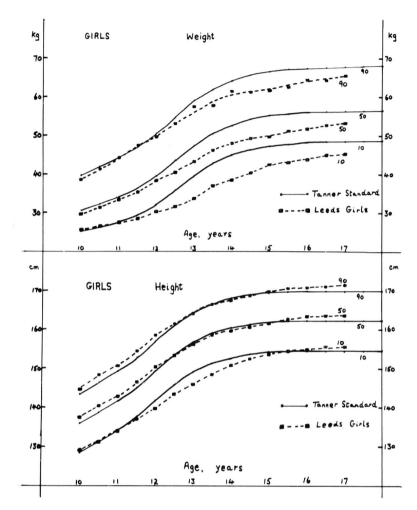

FIGURE 7   Comparison of height and weight centiles in a longitudinal study of 102 Leeds girls and Tanner's 1975 centiles.

Growth standards are continually changing and up to date information is difficult to obtain, but what there is should not be wasted and there is clearly a need to revise growth charts, and to produce norms appropriate for population sub-groups.

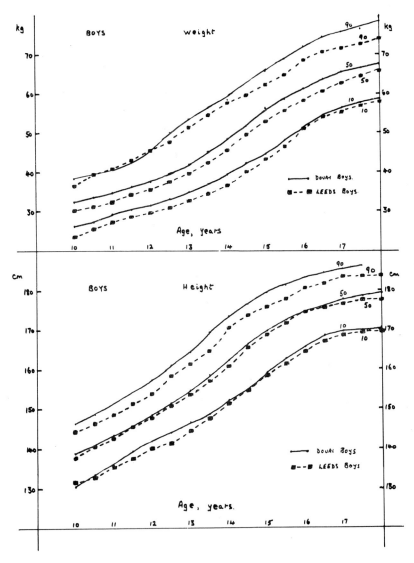

FIGURE 8   Comparison of height and weight centiles in simultaneous longitudinal studies of 96 Leeds schoolboys and 120 boys in a boarding school in Berkshire (Douai).

GROWTH STUDIES IN LEEDS

A longitudinal growth study has recently been completed, and pre-liminary results have been reported. The study commenced in 1973 and has involved undertaking 14 measurements together with pubertal ratings three times per year, i.e. once per term through the years of puberty, on about 100 girls and 100 boys in Leeds day schools. All measurements have been undertaken by me personally and illustrations of the centile spread compared with Tanner's standards are shown in Figures 6 and 7 for boys and girls respectively.

To illustrate the differences in growth patterns of boys from different social and geographical backgrounds and school environments, a simultaneous parallel study has been undertaken on 120 boys at a boarding school in Berkshire (Douai). Figure 8 shows some of the interesting differences between the groups.

These studies provide up-to-date growth information on groups of schoolchildren which can reasonably be compared with those of the Harpenden study, but about 15 years later and from different back-grounds, and illustrate the magnitude of variation that may occur with different population groups in terms of time and setting within the same country.

The Physiology of Growth Hormone Regulation

RICHARD ROSS and MICHAEL BESSER

The Medical College of St. Bartholomew's Hospital, West Smithfield, London EC1A 7BE

The discovery and subsequent synthesis of growth hormone-releasing hormone (GHRH) has greatly advanced our understanding of the factors regulating growth. In this review we have given a brief historical account of the important events leading to the discovery of GHRH, and then discussed the physiology of growth hormone regulation. GHRH, given intravenously, provides a test of the "readily releasable" pool of pituitary GH, but although it can in some cases differentiate hypothalamic from pituitary causes of GH-deficiency, its role as a diagnostic test has not been fully defined. Preliminary studies suggest GHRH may provide an alternative treatment for short stature to GH, and the future development of a long-acting preparation of GHRH may provide an important advance in therapy.

KEY WORDS: Growth hormone, growth hormone-releasing hormone, somatostatin, somatomedins, insulin like growth factor-1

INTRODUCTION

Galen (130–200 AD) was the first to ascribe a function to the pituitary gland. He thought that it was a sump to the brain to which the waste from the conversion of vital spirit to animal spirit drained. It was then excreted from the pituitary, "phlegmatic glandule", as "pituita" or nasal mucus. This view held sway until Richard Lower (1631–1691) disproved the existence of a connection between the brain and naso-pharynx, and suggested that substances pass from the brain to the pituitary and then distilled back into the blood. Although Pierre Marie (1853–1940) reported the connection between acromegaly and an enlargement of the pituitary gland in 1886, he did not recognise this

25

as the cause of acromegaly. It was really Harvey Cushing, in 1909, who first correctly defined the function of the pituitary when he coined the words hyper- and hypo-pituitarism to describe the pathological consequences of hyper- and hypofunction of the pituitary.

Proof that the anterior pituitary contained a growth promoting substance came from studies performed by Herbert M. Evans who demonstrated that the administration of crushed bovine pituitary tissue into rats stimulated somatic growth considerably. Bovine growth hormone was subsequently isolated in 1944, followed by the preparation of a crystalline growth hormone. Although bovine GH promoted growth in a variety of species, it was ineffective in man due to the structural differences between primate and non-primate GH. However, extracted human GH does promote growth, as was first shown by Rabin, who, in 1958, successfully treated a 17-year-old boy with pituitary infantilism and short stature.

The suggestion by Green and Harris, in 1947, that the central nervous system controlled the activity of the pituitary via a neuro-humaral relay, paved the way for the subsequent discovery of the hypothalamic regulatory peptides. In 1960 Reichlin reported that lesions of the ventral hypothalamus in rats decreased the GH content of the pituitary and growth of the animal; demonstrating the importance of the hypothalamus in the control of GH secretion. Further work showed that hypothalamic extracts from rats would stimulate the release of GH from the rat pituitary *in vitro*. Between 1969 and 1981 thyrotrophin releasing hormone, gonadotropin releasing hormone, somatostatin and corticotrophin releasing hormone were isolated from ovine and porcine hypothalmi, although this required vast quantities of animal tissue. For example, between 1964 and 1967, 50 tons of fresh-frozen ovine tissue were processed. Despite the enormous amount of work directed to the discovery of growth hormone-releasing hormone (GHRH), it was not possible to extract it from the animal tissue, because of the small quantities present and the overwhelming amount of somatostatin in the tissue which interfaced with the bioassay. The final characterisation of GHRH in 1982 was exceptional because of its extraction from human tissue, from 2 patients with acromegaly due to the ectopic production of GHRH.

As early as 1960, association between acromegaly and bronchial carcinoid tumours have been noted, and it was subsequently reported that, in similar patients, the acromegaly could be cured by removal of the carcinoid tumour.

In 1980, Dr Michael Thorner of Charlottesville, Virginia, USA, was referred a 21-year-old woman with Turner's syndrome and acromegaly. Histology of pituitary removed by transsphenoidal surgery surprisingly showed somatotroph hyperplasia rather than a pituitary tumour. Subsequent studies revealed that the patient had a pancreatic tumour; the removal of which cured her acromegaly. Portions of the tumour were given to both the groups of Vale and Guilleman. Shortly after this, a similar patient with a pancreatic islet cell tumour was discovered by Dr Sassolas, Lyon, France, and a portion of this tumour was also collected by Guilleman's group. Within one year, the 2 groups of Guilleman and Vale had extracted and sequenced GHRH, and 4 reports of these studies appeared in November 1982.

Extracts from the Lyon tumour showed three forms of GHRH, the longest of which was $GHRH(1-44)NH_2$. Also present were 2 other peptides that were identical in structure, except for shorter length; $GHRH(1-40)OH$ and $GHRH(1-37)NH_2$. The peptide present in the greatest quantity was $GHRH(1-40)OH$. Only one peptide was found in the Charlottesville tumour, which was $GHRH(1-40)OH$. As outlined below, subsequent work has shown that the pancreatic peptides are identical to human hypothalamic GHRH.

The release of GH from the pituitary is under the dual control of 2 hypothalamic hormones; GHRH stimulates and somatostatin inhibits its release (Figure 1). The response to these hypothalamic peptides depends upon both thyroid and steroid hormones. The hypothalamus in turn is influenced by the brain through a complex network of neurotransmitters. GH is released in a pulsatile fashion, with pulses occurring every 3-4 hours, with the greatest release of GH during sleep. There are various physiological stimuli of GH release, and sleep, stress, and exercise account for many of these fluctuations in GH secretion. There is evidence from pharmacological studies that catecholamines, serotonin, histamine, acetylcholine, GABA, and the opiate peptides are involved in the regulation of GH secretion. Growth hormone in turn promotes the synthesis of somatomedin C (SmC), also known as insulin-like growth factor-1 (IGF-1), in the tissues and it is this that is primarily responsible for growth. In the following sections, the evidence for involvement of these various factors in GH secretion is presented.

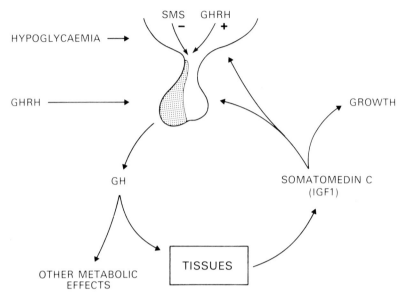

FIGURE 1 The physiology of growth hormone release. SMS = somatostatin, GHRH = growth hormone-releasing hormone, and IGF1 = insulin-like growth factor-1.

GROWTH HORMONE-RELEASING HORMONE

Since the extraction and characterisation of growth hormone-releasing hormone from the pancreatic tumours both 40 and 44 residue peptides identical to these pancreatic peptides have been extracted from several thousand human hypothalamic fragments. GHRH immunostaining has been demonstrated in the arcuate nucleus of the hypothalamus, with fibres projecting to the median eminence and ending in contact with the portal vessels. In addition, the entire human GHRH gene has been structurally characterised and mapped on to chromosome 20. It has been demonstrated *in vitro* that GHRH stimulates transcription of the GH gene as well as GH secretion, and transgenic transfer of the GHRH gene has been shown to increase the growth of mice. Although there has been considerable debate as to which peptide is the native hormone, it is likely that both the 44 and 40 residue peptides are physiologically important.

It appears that the biological activity of GHRH resides principally in the first 29 residues, as analogues of this length with deletions from the C-terminus and retain most of their GH releasing activity, but the N-terminal amino-acid needs to be preserved. Most human studies have been performed with the native peptides or the shorter 29 residue amidated analogues. All 3, when given as an intravenous bolus, selectively promote GH release in normal subjects at doses of 1–3 mcg/kg, although at higher doses such as 10 mcg/kg there may be prolactin release. GHRH potentiates the release of TSH in response to TRH, but has no effect on the responses to the other hypothalamic hormones GnRH and CRH. The only side effect of GHRH reported is facial flushing, which occurs in most subjects within one minute of an intravenous injection, and lasts no longer than 5 minutes.

Subjects aged from 3 days to 86 years have been shown to release GH in response to GHRH. The overall impression is that there is a decreasing GH response to GHRH with age, although there has been some disagreement between studies. Most studies have found no sex difference in response to GHRH, and there is no change in response during the menstrual cycle. GHRH given as an intravenous bolus can be used to define the "readily releasable" pool of GH. It was naturally of great interest to study the responses in growth hormone deficient patients to GHRH, and early studies showed that the majority will release GH in response to an intravenous bolus of GHRH. These patients thus have a defect in either the synthesis or delivery of hypothalamic GHRH, rather than being truly GH-deficient. This finding was not surprising, as a previous post mortem study on a patient with isolated GH deficiency had shown them to have normal pituitary stores of GH. The discovery that GH-deficient children could release GH in response to GHRH suggested that GHRH might provide an alternative treatment to human growth hormone. A number of studies have now reported on the use of GHRH as a therapy for growth hormone deficiency, and it is evident that at least 50% of growth hormone-deficient children will respond to this therapy, given either as twice daily injections or 3 hourly pulses. It is likely that the future development of a depot-preparation of GHRH will provide a major advance in the treatment of GH-deficiency children.

SOMATOSTATIN

The discovery of somatostatin was a biproduct of the search for a

GHRH. In looking for GHRH in rat hypothalmi, a substance that inhibited GH release was unexpectedly detected. This peptide was subsequently extracted from ovine hypothalamic fragments and proved to be a tetradecapeptide. It was called somatostatin, although the name is probably inappropriate as it has many other functions apart from the regulation of GH secretion. Somatostatin is found widely distributed within the nervous system, gut, and endocrine and exocrine glands. It acts both as a neurotransmitter and neuromodulator as well as an endocrine hormone.

There is now ample evidence for a physiological role of somatostatin in the control of GH secretion. The administration of anti-somatostatin antiserum reverses the growth hormone inhibitory effect, and the simultaneous administration of somatostatin blocks the GH response to GHRH. Studies in rats given GHRH after pre-treatment with anti-somatostatin antiserum suggests that there is a tonic secretion of both GHRH and somatostatin into the hypophyseal portal blood, and superimposed onto this there is a 3–4 hourly pulse of GHRH associated with trough levels of somatostatin, resulting in a pulse of GH.

SOMATOMEDIN

The "somatomedin theory" arose from the observation that costal cartilage from hypophysectomised rats was unresponsive to GH added *in vitro*, or to serum from hypophysectomised animals; however it showed marked stimulation and matrix formation in response to normal rat serum. It was hypothesised that there was a "sulphation factor" or "somatomedin" which mediated the effects of GH. Subsequent studies of patients with disorders of the GH-axis showed high levels of sulphation factor in acromegalic patients and low levels in hypopituitary patients, but these rose when patients were given hGH.

Somatomedin peptides have now been isolated from human plasma, and show a very similar structure to insulin, and have therefore also been called insulin-like growth factors. In man, there are 2 distinct chemical forms of the somatomedins; somatomedin-C or insulin-like growth factor 1, and IGF-2. SmC is highly growth hormone dependent, has potent growth promoting activity *in vitro*, and levels reflect GH activity, being high in acromegaly and low in GH-deficiency. The somatomedins, unlike nearly all other peptide hormones, circulate tightly bound to specific serum binding proteins, the physiological significance of which remains unknown. Nevertheless, cartilage and other tissues still respond to somatomedins complexed to binding proteins.

Somatomedins are synthesized by many tissues, including bone, fibrous tissue and the pituitary, although in the adult the liver is probably the greatest source of circulating levels. There has been considerable debate as to whether the somatomedins act as true circulating hormones or whether the principal, important activity lies in the locally produced form which acts in a paracrine or autocrine fashion. Studies infusing GH and SmC into the hind limb of rats have demonstrated a local growth promoting effect which is abolished by antiserum to SmC. Results are consistent with the "somatomedin theory" that the growth promotion action of GH is mediated through SmC, but suggest that the local production is more important in its action.

GROWTH HORMONE FEED-BACK

There is good evidence that GH may modulate its own secretion, but there are few data in man as to the mechanisms involved. It is known that hGH pretreatment attenuates the GH response to pharmacological stimuli, and to physiological stimuli such as sleep and exercise. Recent work has shown that in man that growth hormone pretreatment blocks the growth hormone response to GHRH before circulating levels of IGF-1 have risen. It is therefore evident that GH can autoregulate its own secretion independent of circulating levels of IGF-1, although these may also play a role modulating growth hormone secretion. IGF-1 immunostaining has been demonstrated in the hypothalamus and pituitary, and it may well be that GH feeds-back through the local production of somatomedins at either site. This negative feed back could be mediated either through altered GHRH or somatostatin secretion at the hypothalamus or by a direct effect at the pituitary. Recent work in humans with drugs modulating the cholinergic nervous system, suggest that GH feeds-back through somatostatin, which is under tonic cholinergic control.

Growth hormone feed-back may in part be mediated through other factors apart from GH and SmC; both blood sugar and free fatty acids influence GH release. The administration of free fatty acids or glucose has been shown to attenuate the GH response to GHRH, although it is not clear whether these factors are important in physiological GH release.

THYROID AND STEROID HORMONES

Thyroid hormones, cortisol, and sex steroids all influence GH secretion. Hypothyroidism is associated with decreased GH release, which is corrected by replacement therapy, and similarly in Cushing's syndrome there is deficient GH release with corrects after cure of the disease. In both conditions patients show a poor response to GHRH which reverts to normal when the disease is cured. Oestrogens have an im, ortant influence on GH secretion, and are probably responsible for the difference in GH release between men and women and the change in GH secretion seen during puberty. Most evidence suggests that oestrogens act at the hypothalamus to modulate GHRH release as there seems to be no difference between the sexes or oestrogen status in response to GHRH.

NEUROTRANSMITTERS AND GH RELEASE

Neurons containing catecholamines, acetylcholine, the amino acid neurotransmitter gamma-amino-butyric acid (GABA), and the opioid peptides are found in the hypothalmus. An interaction between these neurotransmitters and somatostatin and GHRH probably leads to pulsatile GH release. Studies with drugs that act as agonists and antagonists at the neurotransmitter receptors allow us to study the physiological relevance of these various neurotransmitters. A full discussion of the role of neurotransmitters in GH secretion is beyond the scope of this review. We have therefore limited ourselves to discussing the role of catecholamines and the cholinergic nervous system.

Depletion of brain catecholamines by alpha-methyl-p-tyrosine sup-presses GH release in the rat, which can be restored by the administra-tion of clonidine, a specific alpha-1 and alpha-2 receptor agonist. The non-selective alpha-adrenergic antagonist phentolamine and selective alpha-2 antagonist yohimbine inhibit GH secretion during insulin-induced hypoglycaemia in healthy young men. Clonidine stimulates GH release in man, and is used as a test of GH secretion. The data available suggest that alpha-2 adrenergic stimulation causes GH release through GHRH as rats depleted in GHRH fail to respond to clonidine. Propranolol, a beta adrenergic blocker, enhances the growth hormone response to insulin-induced hypoglycaemia and GHRH in man. Dopamine stimulates GH release in man, an effect blocked by dopamine agonist; it is likely that the stimulatory action is suprapituitary as dopamine *in vitro* inhibits GH release from the pituitary.

The cholinergic nervous system is important in the regulation of GH secretion. Thus, atropine and pirenzipine, both cholinergic muscarinic antagonists, block the GH response to physiological stimuli of GH secretion, such as sleep and the growth hormone response to GHRH. Similarly, drugs which act by enhancing cholinergic tons such as the acetylcholinesterase inhibitors, increase GH secretion and augment the growth hormone response to GHRH. Data in animals suggest that the effect of cholinergic manipulation on GH secretion is mediated through hypothalamic somatostatin secretion. Acetylcholine inhibits somato-statin release from rat hypothalamus, while the effects of cholinergic manipulation of GH secretion in rats was abolished by hypothalamic somatostatin depletion.

There is a complex interaction between the various transmitters and both somatostatin and GHRH. As yet, it remains unclear as to which peptides and neurotransmitters have an important role in physiological GH secretion.

The last 5 years have seen major advances in our understanding of the factors controlling GH secretion. Many of these discoveries have important clinical implications. It has become increasingly evident that many growth hormone deficient children, rather than having a pituitary defect, have a deficiency either in the synthesis, release or delivery of hypothalamic growth hormone-releasing hormone. This has led to the development of a new therapy with the subcutaneous administration of growth hormone-releasing hormone (Figure 2). It is likely that the future development of a depot-preparation of GHRH will provide a major advance in the treatment of growth hormone deficiency. We are only beginning to understand the importance of the various neuro-transmitters in controlling GH secretion. There has been recent

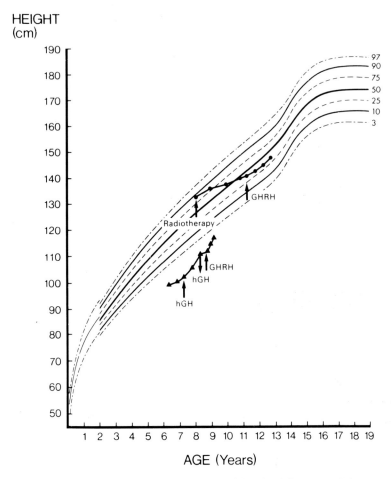

FIGURE 2   Height charts of two boys treated with twice daily sc growth hormone-releasing hormone therapy. (Reproduced with permission from *The Lancet* i: 5–8, 1987).

evidence that some children with GH neurosecretory dysfunction, that is poor physiological release of growth hormone but with normal response to provocative tests, will respond to treatment with drugs which modulate growth hormone secretion at the neurotransmitter level. In particular, a recent study has shown that clonidine will promote growth in some children with neurosecretory dysfunction. It is likely that in the next decade we will see many advances in the treatment and understanding of growth hormone deficiency, and hopefully the development of treatments which will be less intrusive on children's lives as the daily subcutaneous injection of growth hormone.

Epidemiology of Growth Failure

MICHAEL PARKIN

Department of Child Health, The Medical School, Framlington Place,
Newcastle upon Tyne NE2 4HH

KEY WORDS: Short stature, growth hormone deficiency, adult height

Short stature may be a sign of disorder and also a cause of distress to children. Clinicians therefore seek both to prevent growth failure and to treat it whenever possible. In order to provide the necessary service to all children in a community, they need to know the answer to a number of questions and only epidemiological methods are able to provide these.

1. WHAT AFFECTS THE HEIGHTS OF CHILDREN?

In developing countries in all parts of the world there is a marked difference between the heights of children from advantaged homes and those from poor families. The mean heights of children from upper socio-economic groups in these countries are roughly on the 50th centile of growth charts used in developed countries, while the mean heights of children from the lower socio-economic groups are close to the 3rd centile (Figure 1). These differences clearly are the result of the adverse environment associated with disadvantage and indicate the importance of a satisfactory environment for normal growth of children. It seems likely that the main components of the environmental stress in these countries are malnutrition and infection.

The secular trend of an increase in children's heights that has been recorded in several European countries over the last century gives a similar message. Children's growth may be seriously impaired by adverse environment and an increase in their heights therefore is a consequence and an indicator of an improved environment.

37

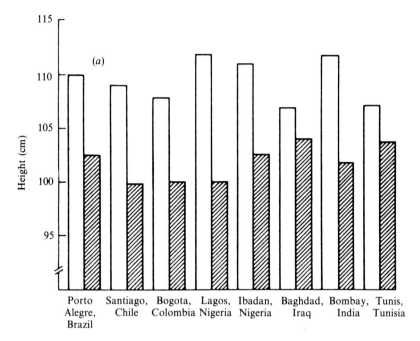

FIGURE 1   Mean heights of 5-year-old boys of upper (open columns) and lower (hatched columns) sodio-economic groups in eight non-European cities. (Reprinted from Eveleth PB, Tanner JM, *Worldwide Variation in Human Growth*, Cambridge University Press, 1976.)

The mean height of ten-year-old boys in England in 1833 was 121 cm, well below the present 3rd centile, that of Swedish boys in 1883 was 130 cm which is on the present 10th centile, while in both countries today it is 140 cm or more (Figure 2). This dramatic increase in children's height has been associated with earlier maturation, most easily measured in girls by age of menarche. As a result the secular trend for adult height has been rather less than that of children, less than 1 cm per decade compared with nearly 2 cm per decade for twelve-year-old children in some societies. Nevertheless, whatever the physiological mechanism, the cause of the secular trend is likely to have been the improved environment in which children live.

In this country, though not in Sweden, there is still a social class gradient in the heights of children. Data published from the National Study of Health and Growth which was started as recently as 1972

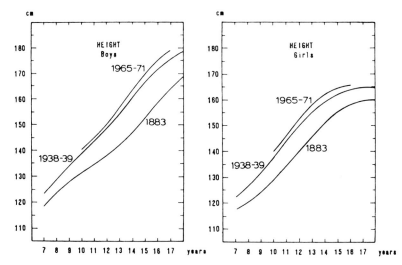

FIGURE 2   Secular trend in growth of height of Swedish boys and girls. (Reprinted from *Annals of Human Biology* 1974; **1**: 245.)

indicated that a decade ago, the five-year-old children of manual workers were 2 cm shorter than those of non-manual workers. This height difference persisted over the next five years of the children's life though it did not increase further.

The relationship between social class and growth in this country is much less pronounced than that seen in developing countries and also is small when compared with the increase in the mean height of children in Europe over the last century. Nevertheless, it indicates that some of our children still live in an environment that is poor enough to restrain their growth. This conclusion raises two questions:

- How important are social variables compared with biological variables in determining the heights of children?

- What is the nature of the environmental defect, related to social class, that leads to growth failure and how does it operate?

Some findings of the 1972 National Study of Health and Growth at first seem to suggest that the effect of environmental influences upon growth, though significant, actually is very small. This study involves about 10 000 children from 28 districts in England and Scotland which

were selected by stratified random sampling, ensuring that proportion-
ately more areas with poorer social groups were included. The effect
of a number of social and biological influences upon the growth of
young children were assessed. It showed, as had previous studies, that
there was a significant relationship between the social variables, sibship
size, father's social class and his employment status and children's
heights, while the most important biological variables affecting height
were the parents' heights and the child's birth weight. However, several
of the variables, both social and biological were interrelated and when
adjustment was made for parental height, the influence of the social
variables on the children's heights diminished. When the data were
analysed to assess the independent effect of each variable, the biological
variables were found to have a much greater effect than the social
variables, although both together accounted for only 30% of the
variance of the children's height (Table I). There remains therefore, the
strong possibility that other unidentified social or environmental
influences are of importance in children's growth.

Although the independent effect on growth of the father's social class
in this study was small, social class should be regarded simply as a
signpost; it only indicates that something in the environment affects
growth. It neither identifies this nor measures its importance. If there
are more important environmental influences affecting growth what
are they?

Under-nutrition is of immense importance in countries in the
developing world but there is little evidence that it is a common cause
of growth failure in this country. A number of studies have indicated

TABLE I

Relationship between social and biological variables and height of children aged 5–11
years

Variable	Percentage of variance of height explained
Social class	0.1
Sibship size	1.28
Employment status	0.05
Birth weight	3.41
Mother's age	0.36
Mother's height	8.39
Father's height	7.05

(Reprinted from Rona RJ, Swan AV, Altman DG, *Journal of Epidemiology and Community Health* 1978; **32**: 147–154.)

that the total food intake of children from poor homes and large families is, in fact, greater than that of children from advantaged homes. This clearly may indicate a difference in the nutritional needs of children being reared in different environments but it also suggests that other causes of growth failure should be sought.

A clue about the nature of such influences upon children's growth was identified in the Newcastle Study of Child Development. In this study, all the children born to Newcastle upon Tyne mothers over three years, 1960–1962, i.e. about 15 000 children altogether, were assessed regularly by health visitors during the first three years of life. They were then measured and had tests of intelligence at the age of five years and again at ten years. Several social variables were shown to affect both the growth and the development of these children but one of the most important was the "care" these children had received during the first three years of life (Figure 3). This was assessed by health visitors

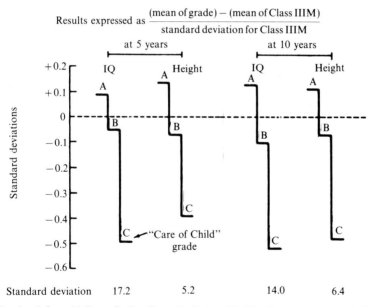

$$\text{Results expressed as } \frac{(\text{mean of grade}) - (\text{mean of Class IIIM})}{\text{standard deviation for Class IIIM}}$$

| Standard deviation | 17.2 | 5.2 | 14.0 | 6.4 |

(Reprinted from Neligan G, Prudham D, Steiner H, *The Formative Years*, Oxford University Press, 1974.)

FIGURE 3   Effect of "Care of Child" grade upon IQ and standardised height at 5 and 10 years in Social Class IIIM (boys and girls).

when the children were three years old in response to the following instructions: "Care of child is intended to include adequacy of food and clothing and of supervision by a responsible adult or older child; cleanliness; seeking appropriate help in case of illness; evidence of affectionate parental interest in the child. If good on all counts, ring A, if poor ring C, if average, ring B." This finding is important and is perhaps a clearer signpost than social class itself, pointing to the real nature of social deprivation. What matters to children is not their social class but how much they are loved and how responsive their parents are to their needs.

Measuring the variables that affect the heights of all children in a society does not necessarily help clinicians who are interested in very short children, especially when growth failure occurs in only a minority of children as it does in this country. Important but special influences affecting the few may be hidden by the common but less relevant influences affecting the majority. To determine the causes of short stature and the relevance to the minority of these studies of the growth of all children, other approaches are necessary.

2. WHAT ARE THE CAUSES OF SHORT STATURE AND HOW COMMON ARE THEY?

Any consideration of the causes of short stature must include the subject of growth hormone deficiency as this is one of the principal conditions in which growth failure is the main problem. Two ways of estimating the prevalence of this have been used. The first is by relating the number of patients diagnosed annually to the number of babies born each year as, in the case of non-fatal conditions beginning in early childhood, prevalence may be equated with birth incidence. This method has disadvantages but it has the great advantage that it can make use of available relevant data without a need for special enquiry. In order to estimate the prevalence of severe growth hormone deficiency the number of applications to the Health Services Human Growth Hormone Committee have been used.

Before 1985, when the only growth hormone available was that derived from human pituitaries, this committee assessed all applications for growth hormone from clinicians in the United Kingdom, and therefore theoretically was informed of every identified patient with growth hormone deficiency. The number of applications to this committee increased steadily until the late 1970s but over the last few years of its work, the number plateaued at about 150 each year. As the annual birth rate in the population at that time was approximately 750 000 these figures suggest that the prevalence of growth hormone deficiency is 1 in 5,000. This may be an underestimate of the true prevalence if some patients suffering from growth hormone deficiency had not been identified. On the other hand, it could be an over estimation as it is based on the number of applications for growth hormone rather than the number of patients who respond to treatment. There is in fact, evidence that 20% of the patients treated with growth hormone at that time were not permanently deficient, as their hormone levels were normal when these were re-tested in adult life. Another and more important reason why this estimate of prevalence might have been too large is that the number of applications was inflated by a back-log of older patients who should have been diagnosed much earlier. When the applications to the Health Services Human Growth Hormone Committee were categorised by year of birth rather than by year of application for treatment, the number of applications fell to about 50 annually, suggesting a prevalence of less than 1 in 10 000.

This technique for estimating the prevalence of individual causes of growth failure not only has the disadvantages already discussed but it is clearly applicable only to conditions that are notified centrally from a large population. It can never be used to identify all the causes or even all the common causes of short stature. This can be determined only by a study of all the short children in a defined population. Such a study obviously is time-consuming because many of the individual causes of short stature are very uncommon and so large numbers of children must be included. However, done properly it can indicate the true prevalence of the conditions defined. The school entry medical examination could be used to provide the relevant information if it were properly co-ordinated as through it data could be available for all children in a community. Sadly, however, with a few exceptions including a current study in Wessex, this potential source of information has not been tapped efficiently.

Data from three studies in the United Kingdom, Newcastle, Scotland and Oxford, however, are available and give information about the causes of short stature.

The Newcastle Study of Child Development was used to collect information about the prevalence of all causes of short stature. The children from the 1960 cohort of births who were still living in Newcastle at ten years of age and had heights at that age under the 3rd centile were studied in detail, together with those from the 1961 and 1962 births who were very short (heights -3 SDs below the mean at that age). Although much detailed data were collected the study was not large enough to determine the prevalence with any degree of certainty of uncommon conditions including severe growth hormone deficiency.

The Scottish study was a much larger one and was designed primarily to determine the prevalence of growth hormone deficiency. Altogether nearly 50 000 schoolchildren aged from 6–9 years from Edinburgh, Aberdeen and Glasgow, the major centres of population in Scotland, were measured and those whose heights were further than 2.5 SDs below the mean of Tanner's standards were examined and investigated.

The most recent study was in Oxford. Its purpose was to evaluate the Oxford Growth Screening Chart which was designed as a means of identifying young children with growth problems. Children starting school in the Oxford health district in 1982 were included and altogether nearly 4,000 of the 6,500 school entrants were screened. Those under the 3rd centile were looked at in detail.

Relevant data from these three studies are shown in Table II.

The objectives of these three studies and the details of the methods and criteria used in them differed, and this accounts for some of the differences. For example, children from special schools with Down's syndrome were not included in the Oxford data. Nevertheless, a number of conclusions may be drawn:

TABLE II
Community studies of short children

Study	Scottish	Oxford	Newcastle
Number measured	48 221	3 864	2 256
Age in years	6–9	5	10
Criterion of abnormality (Tanner standards)	-2.5 SDs	3rd centile	3rd centile
% short children	1%	1.6%	5%
% of short children with organic disease	18%	14%	16%
% of short children with deprivation	31%	6%	30%

- The proportions of children who are short in three parts of the country are very different. There are many more than would be expected from the distribution of Tanner growth centiles in Scotland and the North of England while in Oxford there are fewer.

- The proportions of short children with organic disorders are similar in the three studies. This category includes children with congenital heart disease, cystic fibrosis, chromosomal abnormalities, metabolic disorders, bone disease and mental handicap. However, with the exception of children with Turner's syndrome, other chromosomal abnormalities and growth hormone deficiency, most had been identified and diagnosed before the screening examination in the study.

- The proportion of short children with an underlying organic disorder increases with the severity of the growth failure. Thus in the Newcastle study fewer than 20% of children under the 3rd centile had an organic disease compared with 50% of those whose heights were more than 3 SDs below the mean.

- Amongst those without organic disease a significant number in all areas had evidence of severe psycho-social deprivation. The proportion of deprived children was higher in the North of England and Scotland than in the South though criteria were different. This cause of growth failure may amount to as many as one third of normal short children in some areas.

The data from these community studies are compatible with a prevalence of severe growth hormone deficiency of about 1 in 5,000 children. However, they were carried out before the condition of neuro-secretory endocrine dysfunction was commonly recognised. They therefore are not able to give information about the number of children who need growth hormone because they are physiologically deficient, nor the number who may benefit from growth hormone given for its pharmacological action rather than as replacement treatment. Experience from referral centres suggests that the prevalence of the former group, those with true physiological deficiency or neuro-secretory dysfunction, may be less than that of severe growth hormone deficiency. However, the number of children in these groups depends upon definitions about which as yet there is no agreement, as well as the wider philosophical question about the nature of growth hormone deficiency: Is growth hormone deficiency a specific disorder or is it simply the lower end of the normal distribution of growth hormone production? Further studies of children selected from whole communities are needed to answer this question properly. Nevertheless, clues may be gleaned from an examination of the short normal children in the community studies that have been done.

3. ARE SHORT NORMAL CHILDREN REALLY NORMAL?

Of the 98 children with short stature at 10 years from the cohort of children born in 1960 in the Newcastle study, there were 82 who were described as being short normal. As a group these children had low birth weights and delayed skeletal development and most of their parents were short. In addition, they scored poorly in tests of mental ability and attainment. Many had been reared in poor social circumstances and, as already discussed, it was thought that this had played an important part in causing the short stature in as many as one third.

The level of growth hormone after exercise was measured in all of these children. In two of the most deprived it was low, but in the others the levels were within the range considered normal for provocative tests. The question arises as to whether some of these children had neuro-secretory dysfunction and would have benefitted from growth hormone treatment.

The long-term prognosis of the children may give insights relevant to this question. If children diagnosed as being short normal really had some unrecognised abnormality such a neuro-secretory endocrine dysfunction they may have been expected to have a poor long-term prognosis for height. If, on the other hand, they were really normal, but simply delayed in physical development their final heights would be expected to be satisfactory. We know that delayed development is not an abnormality from data in a much earlier study, the Newcastle Thousand Family Study. In this long-term community study, girls were placed in groups according to the age of their menarche. Those with delayed menarche had the lowest mean height at the age of nine but were taller than average at the age of 22.

Of the 82 short normal children in the Newcastle Study of Child Development whose heights were below the third centile at the age of 10, 50 were traced and re-measured when they were more than 20 years

TABLE III
Longterm prognosis of short normal children

	Male	Female	Both
Total number	25	25	50
Number below 3rd centile as adults	7	10	17
Number >2 cm below 3rd centile as adults	2	1	3
Number taller than predicted	23	11	34
Number >8 cm below target height	1	1	2

old. There was no evidence of any systematic difference in background variables between these 50 and the 32 who could not be traced and so they probably can be taken as representative of the short children in a population of 1500 schoolchildren. There are a number of ways in which their progress can be expressed and these are summarised in Table III.

It can be seen that a minority of the children, though still a significant number, had final heights below the 3rd centile of Tanner charts. Interestingly, the prognosis of those from poor social backgrounds was as good as those who were less deprived. In only three was the height more than 2 inches below the 3rd centile. Clearly the social implications of short stature depend upon an individual's personality, background and aspirations as well as the reactions of society. It can be argued, however, that only three had final heights that might have been a social disadvantage.

The final heights of the children were compared to two other measures, their predicted heights and their expected or target heights. At the age of 11, a prediction of the final heights of the children was made based on height and bone age using the Tanner method. This actually under-estimated the final height of two-thirds of the children rather than the expected one-half.

The other measure with which the final height was compared, was the expected or target height. This was calculated from the measured heights of the parents. All but two of the children had final heights within 8.5 cm of the mid-parental centile, the acceptable range. The two exceptions had heights 8.6 cm and 10.2 cm below the mid-parental centiles.

The fact that virtually all the children had a final height that was within the normal range for their families, of course, does not necessarily mean that they were normal; abnormality may affect more than one generation of a family. However, the finding that no more than three, equivalent to one child in 500 of the initial population, was socially very short is reassuring and perhaps gives some idea of the maximum number of children who may justify growth hormone treatment if it proves to affect the final height of short normal children. The practical question arises as to whether these particular children could have been identified earlier in childhood; but perhaps that is a clinical rather than an epidemiological question! There is at least one difficulty in doing this: growth potential is affected greatly by bone age and in the study described, the shortest adults were not always the shortest children at school.

CONCLUSION

The number of short children in different communities varies, and this variation is largely a result of social differences. In the developing world malnutrition and infection together probably are the major cause of growth failure. In the United Kingdom however, the nature of social disadvantage is less clear but seems to be related to the quality of care received by children. This includes the supply of emotional as well as nutritional needs.

The prevalence of growth hormone deficiency is probably about 1 in 5,000 children but this figure does not indicate the number who should have treatment. However, the long-term prognosis for short children without organic disease, including those who are deprived, is reasonably good. Virtually all have final heights within the normal range for their families and most have heights above the 3rd centile for the community. If treatment in early childhood improves the long-term prognosis for short children and is offered only to those whose final height will be more than 2 inches below the 3rd centile, this may mean 2 children in every 1,000. But perhaps there are better ways of helping children with short stature!

SOURCES OF INFORMATION

Growth of children in the developing world

Eveleth PB, Tanner JM. *Worldwide Variation in Human Growth*. Cambridge University Press, 1976.

Secular trends

Van Wieringen JC. Secular growth changes. In Falkner F, Tanner JM, eds., *Human Growth*, Chapter 16. Bailliere Tindall, London, 1978.
McCullough JM, McCullough CS. Age-specific variation in the secular trend for stature: A comparison of samples from industrialized and nonindustrialized regions. *Am J Physical Anthropology* 1984; **65**: 169–180.

National study of health and growth

Rona RJ, Swan AV, Altman DG. Social factors and height of primary school children in England and Scotland. *J Epid & Comm Health* 1978; **32**: 147–154.
Smith AM, Chinn S, Rona RJ. Social factors and height gain. *Ann Hum Biol* 1980; **7**: 125–128.
Chinn S, Rona RJ. Secular trend in the height of primary school children in England and Scotland 1972–1980. *Ann Hum Biol* 1984; **11**: 1–16.
Rona RJ, Chinn S. Social and biological factors associated with height of children from ethnic groups living in England. *Ann Hum Biol* 1986; **13**: 453–471.

Scottish growth study

Vimpani GV. *et al.* Prevalence of severe growth hormone deficiency. *Brit Med J* 1977; **ii**: 427–430.
Vimpani GV. *et al.* Differences in physical characteristics, perinatal histories and social background between children with growth hormone deficiency and constitutional short stature. *Arch Dis Child* 1979; **56**: 922–928.

Oxford growth data

Aynsley-Green A, Macfarlane JA. Method for early recognition of abnormal stature. *Arch Dis Child* 1983; **53**: 535–537.
Macfarlane A, Ahmed L, Aynsley-Green A. Screening for stature at school entry using the Oxford growth screening chart. (Unpublished). 1985.

Newcastle study of child development

Neligan G, Prudham D, Steiner H. *The Formative Years.* Oxford University Press, 1974.
Lacey KA, Parkin JM. The normal short child. *Arch Dis Child* 1974; **49**: 417–424.
Lacey KA, Parkin JM. Causes of short stature: A community study of children in Newcastle upon Tyne. *The Lancet* 1974; Jan. 12: 42–45.
Neligan G, Prudham D. Family factors affecting child development. *Arch Dis Child* 1976; **51**: 853–858.
Lacey KA, Parkin JM. Long term prognosis for short normal children. (Unpublished data).

Newcastle thousand family study

Miller FJW, *et al. Growing up in Newcastle upon Tyne.* Oxford University Press, London, 1960.
Miller JFW, Billewicz WZ, Thomson AM. Growth from birth to adult life of 442 Newcastle upon Tyne schoolchildren. *Brit J Prev Soc Med* 1972; **26**: 224–230.

The Clinical Spectrum

PETER BETTS

Level C, East Wing, Southampton General Hospital, Southampton SO9 4XY

Accurate measurements of height and the calculation of height velocity should be determined in children of short stature together with the mid-parental height centile. Non-endocrine causes of short stature include chromosomal, genetic and intra-uterine abnormalities. Following birth, emotional deprivation is an important factor in short stature but nutritional causes and disorders of the gut and the kidneys should be considered.

Hypothyroidism and Cushings syndrome together with excess steroid dosage for systemic disorders should also be considered together with the possibility of growth hormone deficiency.

KEY WORDS: Short stature, growth velocity, non-endocrine and endocrine factors

What is short stature? There can be no doubt that the child in Figure 1 is small. At the age of three she weighed four kilograms and was only 60 centimetres tall, well below the third centile. She has a rare syndrome leading to extreme short stature. What of the five-year-old in Figure 2 whose height lies on the third centile: is he small in stature? If his father's height were on the tenth centile and his mother on the third then, by these criteria, his height would be appropriate to his genetic background. If, on the other hand, the height of his parents lay in the upper centiles, he would be considered inappropriately small. Whether a child's height is appropriate or otherwise is important, but not nearly as important as the growth velocity where the real definition of normality lies.

In the simplest terms, normal children grow between the 75th and the 25th centiles for velocity. Growth velocity should be measured over a 12 month period because of the error involved in measuring over a

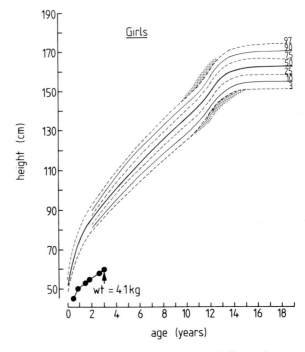

FIGURE 1   Short stature due to Kenny–Caffey syndrome.

shorter period. Multiplying up a six-month velocity to gain the annual growth rate can lead to serious error. If the height velocity lies persistently below the 25th centile, the chances are high of finding a pathological (but often remediable) cause. The child on the 3rd centile for height will fall away from it if his velocity is below the 25th centile.

The boy in Figure 3 has Down's syndrome. Children with chromosomal disorders are often short in stature but that fact does not preclude them from having another abnormality responsible for their short stature which might be remediable. There is, for example, an increased frequency of hypothyroidism in people with Down's syndrome. At the age of four years this child's height lay at six standard deviations below the mean of normals for that age. Careful investigation, however, also revealed pituitary hypothyroidism and growth hormone deficiency. Prior to treatment with growth hormone, he was growing at three

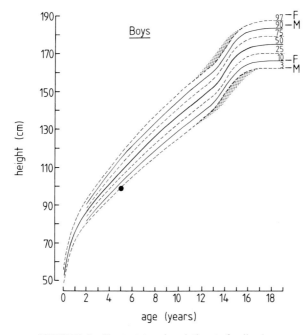

FIGURE 2   Short stature in relation to family size.

centimetres per year (Figure 4) and falling away from his peers. Indeed, had he remained unrecognised and untreated, he would barely have been able to sit on the chair at his desk on school entry the following year. The growth acceleration following treatment is clear from the graph. It is therefore important to realise that the presence of one condition known to cause small stature does not preclude the presence of others.

The girl in Figure 5 has Turner's syndrome, with webbing of the neck, widely spaces nipples, wide carrying angle, delayed puberty and short stature. Not all cases of Turner's syndrome are quite so easy to diagnose. While a group of Turner's children often look typical, the individual case diluted by many other conditions in a busy paediatric clinic may be missed. The paediatrician must check the chromosomes of every slowly growing girl and recognise that some may have Turner mosaicism. Another important point to remember in the early recog-

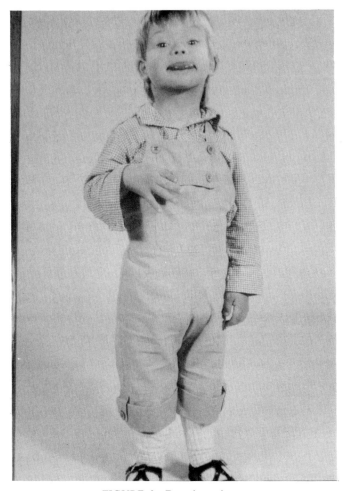

FIGURE 3   Down's syndrome.

nition of Turner's syndrome is the lymphoedema of the lower limbs sometimes present in the newborn. Although the response of Turner's children to growth hormone is at present uncertain (though encouraging), early recognition is important to provide the opportunity of counselling both child and parents through the early years. The questions of puberty, breast development, etc., can then be broached well in advance. The chart in Figure 6 shows that some 50% of young

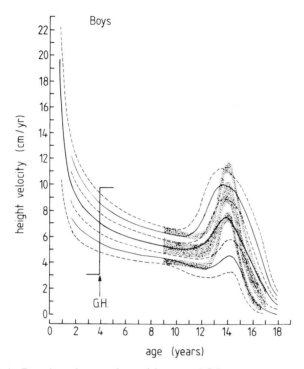

FIGURE 4   Down's syndrome and growth hormone deficiency – response to treatment.

Turner's children will lie within the normal centiles for height. The problem arises when, from school entry age onwards, growth velocity falls and with it the height of the child relative to her peers. It is, therefore, vitally important to measure at serial intervals the height of the child whose mother at school entry thinks she is growing slowly. There is nowadays a much increased awareness of the appropriate hormonal replacement for children with Turner's syndrome using low-dose oestrogens and perhaps growth hormone. There is a growing literature on the subject, indicating the use of small doses of oestrogen from an early age, and certainly from eight or nine years.

   Noonan's syndrome has features similar to Turner's syndrome. Figure 7 shows the wide carrying angle. Often there is low intelligence and associated congenital heart abnormalities. The outward and downward slanting of the eyes, typical of Noonan's syndrome, may

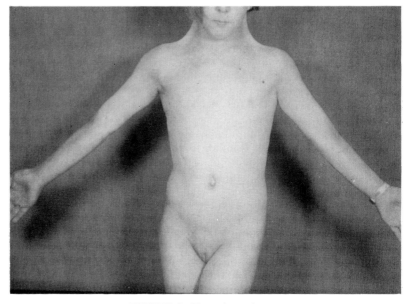

FIGURE 5   Turner's syndrome.

also be seen. Noonan's syndrome is not a chromosomal abnormality but, like Turner's children, Noonan's children grow slowly.

Turning from chromosomal to genetic disorders, Figure 8 is a reminder that the proportions of the body change with age such that in adulthood the level of the symphysis pubis represents about half total height whereas at birth the level of the umbilicus represents about half total length. Genetic disorders which affect development of the trunk will inhibit height as will disorders affecting the growth of the limbs (e.g. achondroplasia). The young boy in Figure 9 shows an extreme form of achondroplasia, with short stature and marked disproportion. The child in Figure 10 has a form of pseudoachondroplasia with a relatively large head in proportion to the body and a disproportionately low symphysis pubis on account of his short limbs. There is currently promising work going on in the area of orthopaedic bone lengthening to help children with these conditions. An acquired form of trunk disproportion, which must not be forgotten is that resulting from spinal irradiation in cases of a medulloblastoma.

Intrauterine environment exerts a major influence on subsequent

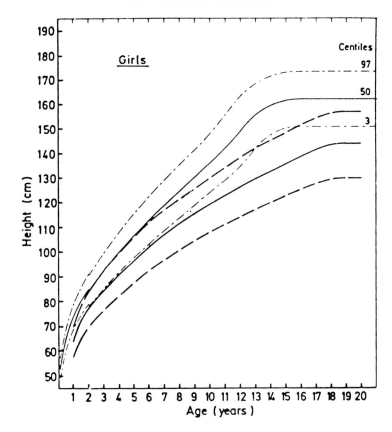

*Mean height (2 SD) at different ages calculated
from published data on patients with Turner syndrome*

FIGURE 6   Growth chart for girls with Turner's syndrome (published with kind
permission from Castlemead Publications).

growth. Figure 11 shows a child with Russell–Silver syndrome, a child
of low birth weight, though perhaps normal gestation, who may have
skeletal disproportion with one side of the body being rather smaller
than the other (in this case the left smaller than the right) and a
somewhat triangular face.

Extrauterine environment during the formative years strongly influences growth velocity and ultimate height. The young girl depicted

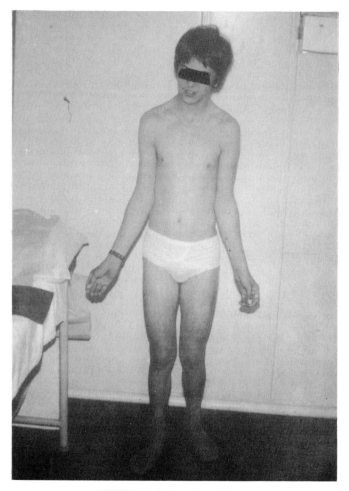

FIGURE 7   Noonan's syndrome.

in Figure 12 was unhappy in a children's home in New York with the typical features of emotional deprivation, such as radar-like gaze and constant anticipation of what was going on around her. When removed from the home to a happier environment she grew rapidly, filled out and looked much more alert and content. This is the syndrome of emotional or psychosocial deprivation. Not all children show such

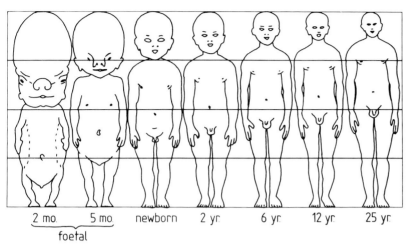

FIGURE 8   Changes in body proportion.

obvious features but most paediatricians will be aware of the child, such as the example in Figure 13, taken into the care of a foster home whereupon growth accelerated rapidly. At present we have no idea what proportion of the childhood population is growing suboptimally as a result of the psycho-social syndrome. It is also unclear whether the primary cause of short stature in emotional deprivation is hormonal or concurrent nutritional deprivation. There is no doubt, however, that, while unhappy, such children have suppressed growth hormone release and that when taken into a happier environment for a period of time, will normalise their growth hormone release profile. A means to distinguish between the nutritional and emotional components in psychosocial deprivation syndrome will bring an important advance to our understanding of depressed growth in childhood.

Gastroenterological causes of short stature are often very difficult to unravel in the clinical situation. The two girls in Figure 14 are of the same age. The one admitted to hospital for minor surgery, the other for investigation of short stature, rickets, pallor and misery. The latter, with her pot belly and wasted buttocks, is a case of coeliac disease. The growth velocity is often very low and responds rapidly to a gluten free diet. The child represented in Figure 15 was screened on school

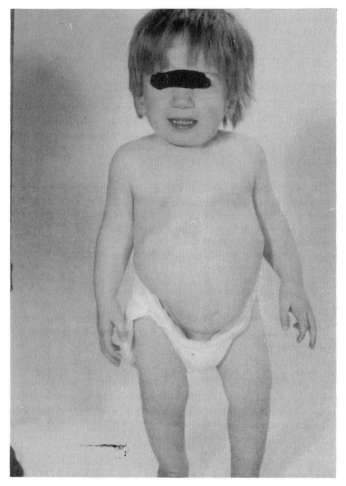

FIGURE 9   Achondroplasia.

entry at the age of five, was noted to be on the third centile and, because she was "normal", was not followed further. She was entirely asymptomatic until she presented again at the age of 12 with short stature, this time well below the third centile, a haemoglobin of 78 g per litre and an iron deficiency picture. A jejunal biopsy showed total villous atrophy. On a gluten free diet, the growth accelerated. The lesson to

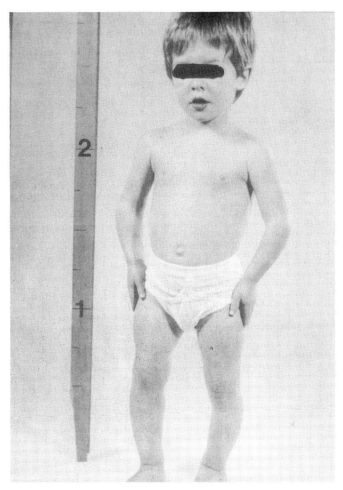

FIGURE 10   Pseudoachondroplasia.

be learned from this child is that gluten enteropathy may be entirely asymptomatic.

Another nutritional complaint responsible for slow growth in short stature is cystic fibrosis. Figure 16 shows the fat globules in the stool of a cystic child. Although it is unlikely that a child would be missed, recurrent chest infections and failure to thrive should provide the necessary diagnostic clues. Remaining with the gastrointestinal system,

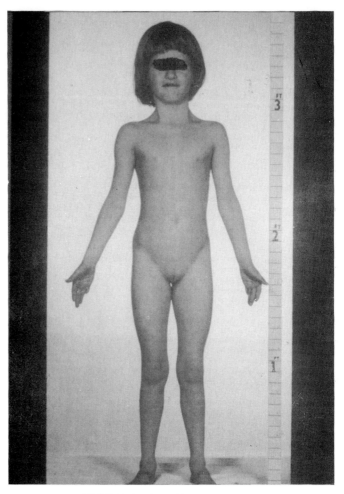

FIGURE 11   Russell–Silver syndrome.

the young girl of eight in Figure 17 presented with apthous ulcers and anaemia. She was investigated for coeliac disease but had a normal jejunal biopsy. A barium meal and follow through were normal at that time, although the ESR was 24 mm per first hour. She was followed for a short time afterwards, her height fell across the centiles but she failed to re-attend for follow-up. By the age of eleven-and-a-half years,

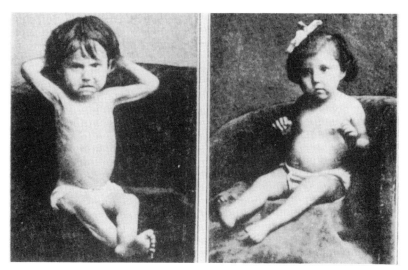

FIGURE 12   Emotional deprivation before and after treatment.

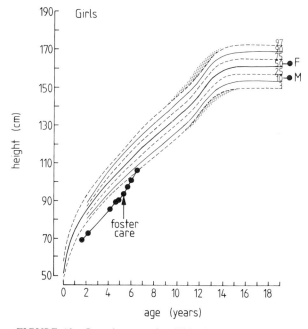

FIGURE 13   Growth curve of a child taken into foster care.

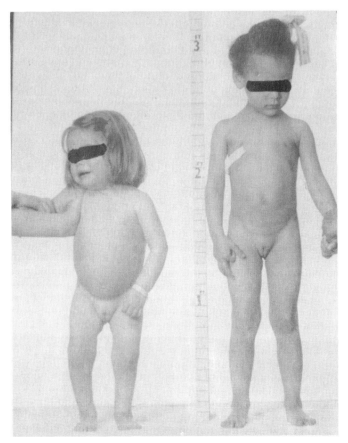

FIGURE 14   Girl on the left has coeliac disease compared with a child of normal height.

he height was now below the 3rd centile, the ESR 44 mm per first hour, the haemoglobin 90 g per litre and the barium follow through now showed the typical string pattern of Crohn's disease of the terminal ileum. She had been complaining of intermittent abdominal pain during recent years, general tiredness and misery, but no blood or mucus in the stools. Crohn's disease is an important and often undiagnosed cause of small stature and should be considered particularly in a child who is anaemic or who has an unexplained fall off in growth velocity (i.e.

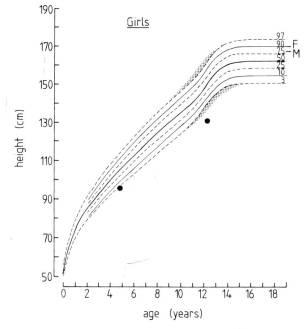

FIGURE 15   Growth curve of late onset of coeliac disease.

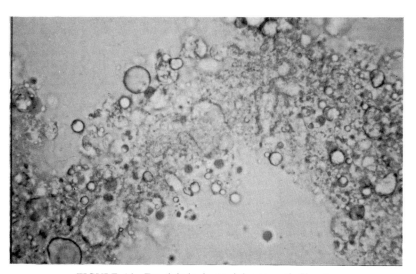

FIGURE 16   Fat globules in stool due to cystic fibrosis.

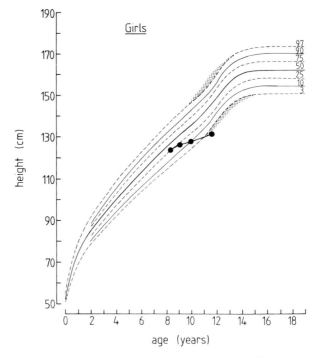

FIGURE 17   Growth curve of girl with Crohn's disease.

crosses the height centiles). It may otherwise remain occult for many years.

The child in Figure 18 presented to the general practitioner with a story of polydipsia and polyuria going back many years. His creatinine was rising steadily and he was on a dialysis programme for chronic renal failure within two years of being seen. He was suffering from congenital nephronophthisis. Although this is a rare presentation, short stature is a recognised feature of chronic renal failure. The typical pattern of growth in children with kidney failure is shown diagrammatically in Figure 19. Children with congenital renal abnormalities are smaller than those with acquired abnormalities, as they often fail to thrive during the first years of life. Difficulty in feeding, biochemical disturbance and problems with vomiting all play a role. The need for ensuring adequate nutrition in such children recognised as "at risk" from the start cannot be overemphasised. With maturation of kidney

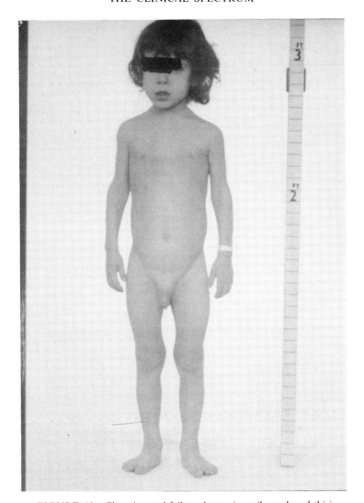

FIGURE 18   Chronic renal failure due to juvenile nephrophthisis.

function and stabilising of their condition, the children with chronic renal failure will often grow normally throughout childhood until the onset of terminal renal failure with its attendant osteodystrophy. Of recent interest are the observations from a Los Angeles group that the poor growth velocity of children with chronic renal failure can be improved with growth hormone administration, so that it may be

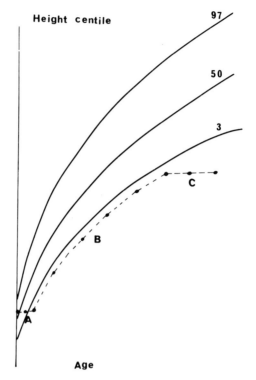

FIGURE 19   Growth pattern of children with chronic renal failure commencing in infancy.

possible to help them during the period of renal failure prior to dialysis and/or transplantation. Figure 20 dates back to 1918 and shows a child with gross osteodystrophy. Renal osteodystrophy becomes important as the glomerular filtration rate falls below $30 \, ml/min/1.73^2$. Vitamin D and phosphate binders are given, where appropriate, to deal with the hypocalcaemia secondary to hyperphosphataemia.

The smaller of the two friends in Figure 21 has Bartter's syndrome, an abnormality associated with electrolyte losses from the renal tubules. There are increased quantities of prostaglandins in the urine and (probably secondary) hypertrophy of the juxtaglomerular apparatus. Why should these children fail to grow? Is it their metabolic electrolyte imbalance or is it failure to take sufficient calories? A point of practical

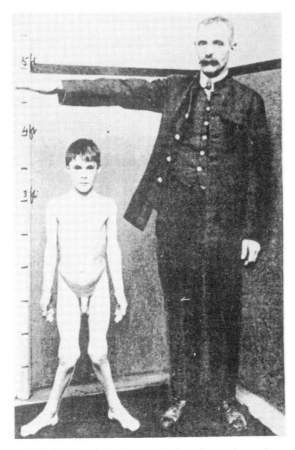

FIGURE 20   Old photograph of renal osteodystrophy.

importance is the considerable improvement in growth velocity following potassium supplementation and prostaglandin synthetase inhibitors
in the form of indomethacin. Figure 22 shows the sort of response that
can be expected.

Finally, let us turn to the hormonal causes of short stature. The
patient in Figure 23 presented when four years of age and had not
grown for the previous two years. Hypothyroidism was diagnosed and
treatment with thyroxine led to an acceleration of growth and change
in appearance (Figure 24). Hypothyroidism in young children is often

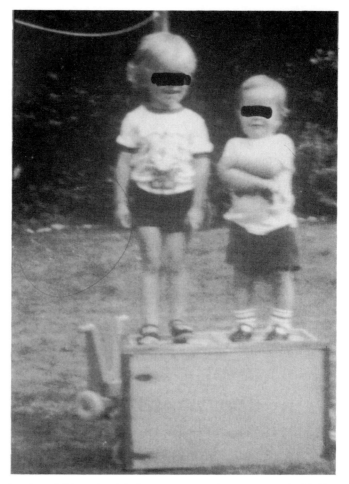

FIGURE 21 Child on the right har Bartter's syndrome compared with his normal friend.

difficult to diagnose. Small, fat children should always be considered with this diagnosis in mind, one important alternative being growth hormone deficiency.

The two girls in Figure 25 presented at the age of 14 within about four months of each other. Neither had grown since the age of eight and it had taken this length of time to present to the growth clinic. Families, as a whole, are not so worried about small girls as they are

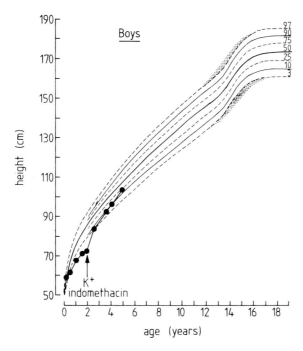

FIGURE 22 Growth pattern of child with Bartter's syndrome treated with indomethacin and potassium.

about small boys. There are many more boys referred for problems of small stature and many more boys than girls on growth hormone treatment at any one time. This is perhaps a reflection of society's interest rather than any sex difference in pathology. The two girls in Figure 25 complained of small stature, thin hair, sallow features and dry skin. One had also had precocious breast development and began menstruating before the appearance of pubic hair. A functional increase in FSH secretion parallel with the rising TSH secretion is well known to occur in primary thyroid failure. The girl in Figure 26 was also suffering from hypothyroidism. At the age of six/seven years she was tall but her father's height lay above the 97th centile. She was followed up but, although her mother kept claiming that she was failing to grow, none of the medical attendants she saw connected the heights together to reveal the dramatic fall across the centiles which she was experiencing. Eventually, her weight was on the 97th centile, but her height on the

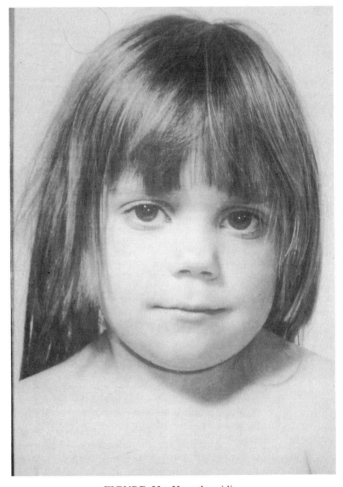

FIGURE 23   Hypothyroidism.

10th centile. This, again, illustrates how important the rate of growth is compared with height attained. It may take a long period of years for a child who is growing nevertheless very poorly to fall from the 97th to the 3rd centile for height. Use of the height centiles as a definition of normality make a nonsense in these circumstances.

Thyroid autoantibodies are a useful means of screening for thyroiditis and Professor Deborah Doniach showed many years ago that approxi-

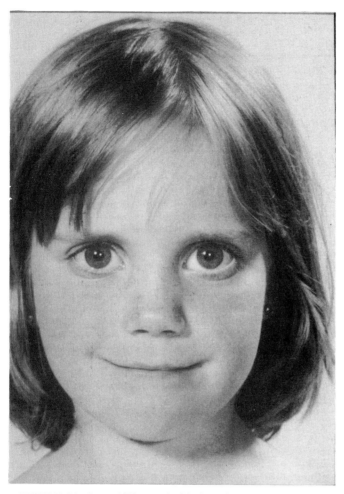

FIGURE 24   Same child treated with thyroxine for hypothyroidism.

mately 2% of children under the age of ten were positive for thyroid autoantibodies and 4% of young people under the age of 20. This does not mean that all are going to develop hypothyroidism, but all should be considered at risk and their growth development and thyroid function checked regularly. Autoimmune thyroiditis is much commoner in girls than in boys and is frequently familial, emphasising the

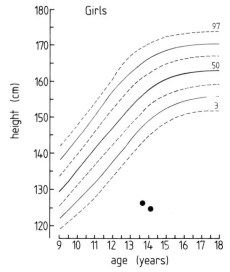

FIGURE 25   Growth chart of two adolescents presenting with hypothyroidism.

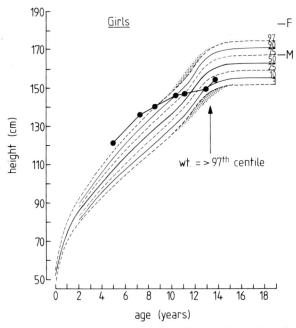

FIGURE 26   Growth chart of girl with undiagnosed hypothyroidism.

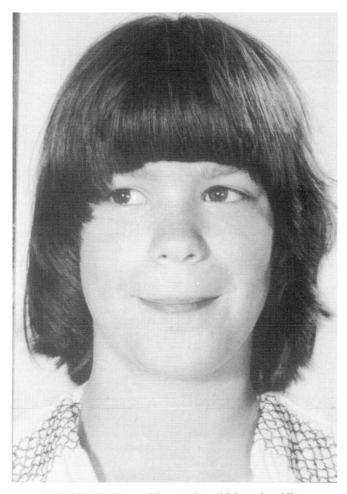

FIGURE 27   Young girl presenting with hypothyroidism.

importance of family history. The young lady in Figure 27 presented with poor growth and early breast development. Her mother was already on thyroxine for hypothyroidism and her sister had goitrous hypothyroidism as well. It is important to bear in mind the other clinical associations of hypothyroidism, which reflect an underlying autoimmune diathesis. The child in Figure 28 had diabetes diagnosed

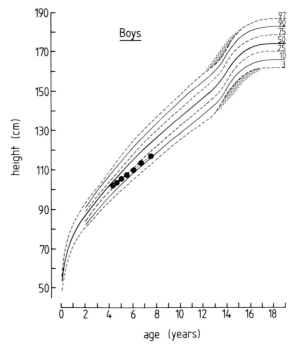

FIGURE 28   Growth pattern of a boy with diabetes and acquired hypothyroidism.

at the age of four and also suffers from asthma. He had been monitored for over 12 months in the belief that his poor growth was related to poor control of his diabetes but, on testing, his serum free thyroxine was found to be 1.6 pg/l and the TSH 68 mu/l, typical of severe primary hypothyroidism.

The young man in Figure 29 was attending infrequently on account of a sacral spina bifida diagnosed at birth. However, although he started to enter puberty, his growth and development appeared to slow down and his growth chart (Figure 30) showed how he had fallen from his usual centile. While his peers were undergoing a growth spurt during early puberty, this patient was doing the reverse. He had childhood Cushing's disease which is particularly difficult to recognise. Unfortunately, he was well into puberty by the time the diagnosis was confirmed and there was little potential for further growth. His height ended up at 150 centimetres. The situation in Figure 31 is hopefully preventable.

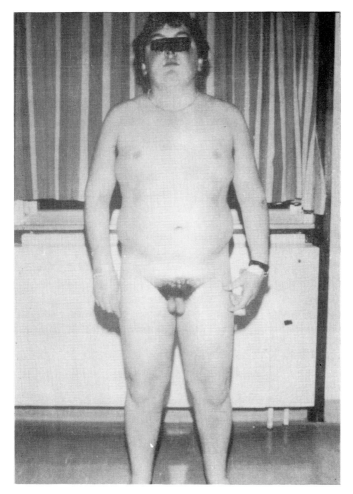

FIGURE 29   Adolescent with Cushing's syndrome.

She is around 140 centimetres in height, grossly Cushingoid and had been treated repeatedly with dexamethasone since she was eight for asthma. Steroids suppress growth.

Finally, to return to growth charts and their proper usage. The young lad represented in Figure 32 was measured on several occasions from the age of five. Had one simply repeated his height at the age of six

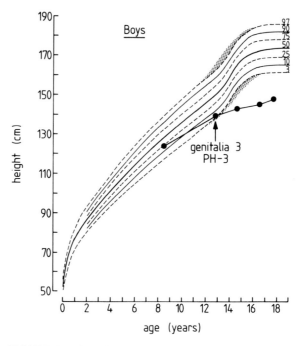

FIGURE 30   Growth pattern of boy with Cushing's syndrome.

and plotted the result on a high distance chart, it is likely that
his problem would have gone undetected because the scale is so small.
Only in subsequent years does it become apparent that the serial plots
are falling progressively across the centiles. The scale on a velocity
chart is much larger, so that poor growth velocities or growth velocities
which change over a short period of time can be detected immediately.
It cannot be too often repeated that to stay on the 3rd centile for height,
a child must have a mean height velocity at the 25th centile. A
child growing at the 3rd centile for growth velocity will fall away
progressively from his height centile. Screening at appropriate times
during childhood, accurate measurement of height and the proper
monitoring of the results, are basic to preventative health care in
childhood. At this point in time, too little attention is paid to this
aspect of child care and many errors of omission are being made. It is
hoped that the simple principles laid down in this chapter may reduce
them.

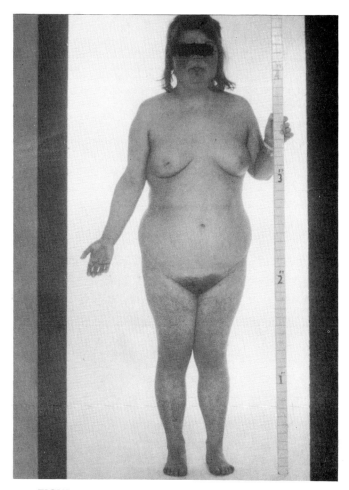

FIGURE 31   Adolescent with iatrogenic Cushing's syndrome.

PETER BETTS

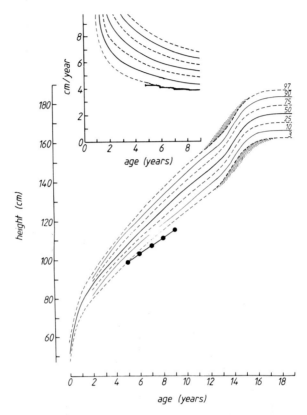

FIGURE 32   Growth chart showing longitudinal growth and growth velocity of a boy with growth hormone deficiency.

Growth Hormone Therapy

C. G. D. BROOK

Endocrine Unit, The Middlesex Hospital, Mortimer Street, London W1N 8AA

The term growth hormone deficiency should be restricted to children who have deletion of the GH gene. GH secretion is otherwise continuous from very small children growing very slowly to very tall children who become tall by growing quickly. Any child given growth hormone will grow more quickly but the prognosis for final height is determined by growth status or the start of treatment and the vigour with which treatment is applied.

KEY WORDS: Growth, growth hormone, growth hormone treatment

It is now well recognised that there is a substantial difference in the amount of growth hormone secreted by tall children compared with small children. However, a real difficulty in interpreting 24 hour profile studies stems from the lack of any cut-off with which to define normality. Just as you cannot define obesity at a particular skinfold thickness, so there is a continuum of growth hormone secretion between two extremes, with every gradation represented. In one sense, the Growth Hormone Committee did a disservice by applying an arbitrary cut-off to "normal" growth hormone levels which has shaped thinking and misdirected ideas about the use of growth hormone in an unfortunate way, even though, at the time, such restriction was necessary to limit demand for a substance available in limited amounts. In some respects we are at the stage with growth hormone which corresponds to the first use of cortisone in the treatment of Addison's disease: cortisone was lifesaving in physiological doses in Addison's disease but equally lifesaving in asthma and transplant therapy at very different doses. We need now to explain the full therapeutic potential of growth hormone.

Figure 1 shows the 24 hour growth hormone profiles of four children on 3rd centile for height growing at 50th, 10th, 3rd centile velocities either with GH responses to insulin induced hypoglycaemia. It can be seen that in these children growth velocity is reflected both in 24 h GH profiles and in GH responses to insulin induced hypoglycaemia. This consonance is not invariable. Figure 2 shows a good GH response to insulin induced hypoglycaemia but hopelessly disordered GH secretion.

This disorganised pattern of GH release has been called neuro-secretory dysfunction. Its definition is difficult and it affects relatively few children, but mention of it does serve to point out the fundamental flaw in all the studies investigating the use of growth hormone in so-called normal children defined solely by their response to insulin induced hypoglycaemia. The simpler tests confirm the secretion profile most of the time, but sometimes they mislead and they are certainly not a gold standard.

Overall, it is well established that the amount of growth hormone secreted by a child relates to the rate at which he grows.[1] Figure 3 shows this relationship in 50 short prepubertal children. The lower asymptote (B) shows the rate at which a child will grow if he has no growth hormone secretion, which may result from a deletion of the growth hormone gene. The rate of growth in the presence of unlimited growth hormone is shown by the upper asymptote (A). In this particular study the dimension of A approaches zero but it must actually enter the positive range in a normal population because otherwise tall children would not exist and nor would pituitary giants. It should be noted that the variables are continuous on both axes and the graph reveals a lot about the effects of growth hormone given therapeutically. The administration of small amounts of growth hormone to very slowly growing children will result in a considerable increase in growth rate. To obtain the same increase in growth rate for a child who is growing less slowly would require a much greater amount of growth hormone. The more growth hormone administered, the more the effect but the question of dose and frequency of administration is complex. The message however is clear: any child given growth hormone will grow more rapidly, including normal children.[2]

If the asymptotic regression between height velocity and GH secre-tion is correct, the pre-treatment rate of growth or the pre-treatment growth hormone secretory status will predict the response to a given amount of growth hormone. Figure 4 shows this to be the case. The UK, uniquely in the world, held rigidly to the notion that there was a standard dose of growth hormone which all children needed. This has meant that we have treated very small children with a lot of growth

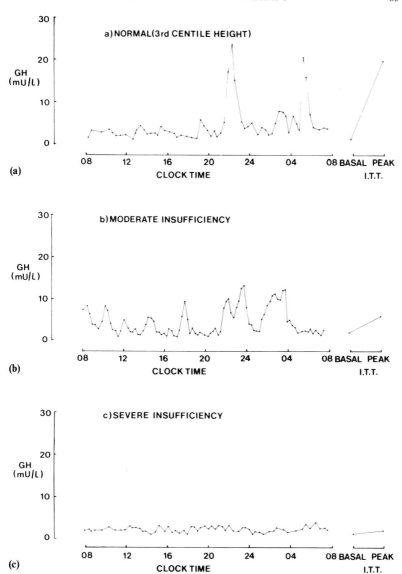

FIGURE 1   24 hour growth hormone profiles of children 3rd centile for height growing at (a) 50th centile, (b) 10th centile, (c) 3rd centile velocities together with GH responses to insulin-induced hypoglycaemia.

CHARLES BROOK

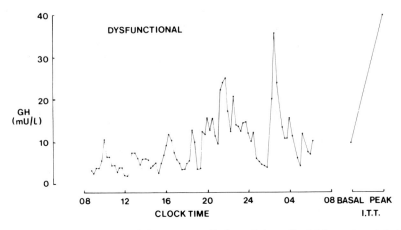

FIGURE 2   24 hour growth hormone profile from 3rd centile child growing at 3rd centile velocity due to neurosecretory dysfunction. Note brisk response to insulin-induced hypoglycaemia.

hormone and larger children with relatively little, amounts often quite inappropriate for their needs. In trying to derive some useful data about the dose and effect from these observations, Figure 5 shows the lines of best fit for children who were treated on a dose of growth hormone greater or less than 15 units/M^2/week. Dose makes little difference to the child growing very slowly because he experiences a considerable increase in velocity with a small amount of growth hormone. But the GH required to maintain that response in children growing at a more normal height velocity increases greatly. Finally, in Figure 6 are shown the effects of frequency of hormone administration on response.[3]

   Our studies clearly show that any child given growth hormone will grow more quickly. But this begs the question whether the acceleration in growth will actually be of benefit in the long term. The therapeutic nihilist will say there is no point in treating a child if it makes no difference to the ultimate height achieved, but I do not side with him. Consideration must be given to the child of 16 who has delayed puberty, who is growing slowly, is getting left behind, has been thrown out of the Colts 15, and is faced with his GCSE but beginning to fail academically because he feels a social reject. Even his university

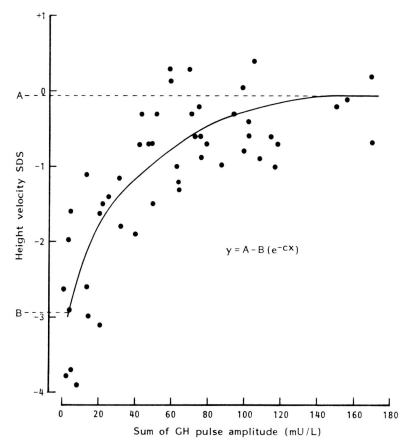

FIGURE 3   The relationship between height velocity standard deviation score for chronological age and sum of growth hormone pulse amplitudes in 50 short prepubertal children.

interview may be influenced by his immature appearance. I believe that such a child needs treatment for his social circumstances, even if studies show that there is no benefit in the longer term.

Some of our own experience with the long term use of pituitary growth hormone is shown in Figure 7.[4] Here are shown height standard deviation scores of 58 children prepubertal at the start of growth

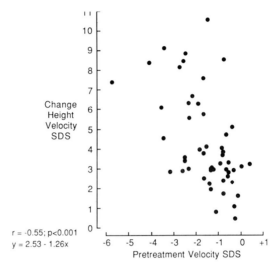

FIGURE 4   Change in height velocity standard deviation score for chronological age following treatment with biosynthetic human growth hormone for 1 year compared to pre-treatment height velocity standard deviation score.

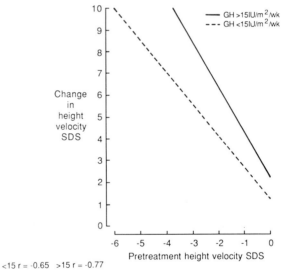

FIGURE 5   Legend as for Figure 4. The relationship of dose to change in height velocity.

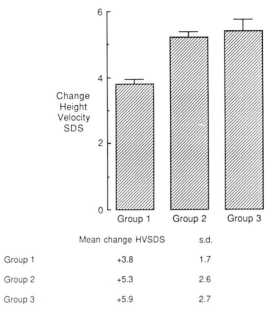

Mean change HVSDS		s.d.
Group 1	+3.8	1.7
Group 2	+5.3	2.6
Group 3	+5.9	2.7

FIGURE 6   Effect of frequency of change in height velocity after treatment with biosynthetic human growth hormone. Group 1 received 4 units of growth hormone 3 times/week, Group: 2 units of growth hormone 6 times/week, Group 3: 1 unit of growth hormone 12 times/week.

hormone treatment and prepubertal throughout five years of continuous treatment with growth hormone. Pre-pubertal status is important because puberty makes growth analysis very difficult. There was progressive improvement in growth but the height SDS for bone age, which predicts ultimate height, was the same at the end of treatment as it was at the start. This does not mean that the growth hormone was without effect, because if the children had not been treated, and had continued to grow very slowly, their height standard deviation score for chronological age would have fallen steadily and their bones would eventually fuse with a much reduced final height. Thus growth hormone prevents further deterioration of height potential. Corresponding data for puberty show curves which converge because a child pubertal at the start of treatment will very soon match bone age with

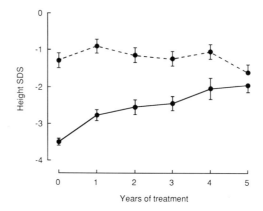

FIGURE 7   Height SDS for chronological age (dotted line) and for bone age (solid line) for 58 children prepubertal throughout the course of 5 years of treatment with pituitary growth hormone.

chronological age as epiphyses fuse. Such children will obviously do less well in the end than the children treated prepubertally.

In conclusion, any child given growth hormone will grow more quickly. Growth hormone will maintain normal growth in growth hormone deficient subjects but the prognosis for the final height is determined by the growth status when therapy is started and the vigour with which the therapeutic regimen is applied. Doses of growth hormone need to be tailored for size and given by daily subcutaneous injection.

References

1. Hindmarsh P, *et al.* The relationship between height velocity and growth hormone secretion in short prepubertal children. *Clin Endocrinol* 1987; **27**: 581–591.
2. Hindmarsh PC, Brook CGD. Effect of growth hormone on short normal children. *Br Med J* 1987; **295**: 573–577.
3. Smith PJ, Brook CGD. Therapeutic alternatives: GHRH or GH treatment in GH insufficiency? *Arch Dis Child* (in press).
4. Bundak R, Hindmarsh PC, Smith PJ, Brook CGD. Longterm auxological effects of human growth hormone (hGH). *J Pediatr* (in press).

Growth at Puberty

MARTIN SAVAGE

Department of Child Health, St. Bartholomew's Hospital, West Smithfield, London EC1A 7BE

Growth at puberty is an important component of normal linear growth. The adolescent growth spurt (AGS) is the result of a critical concentration of sex steroids combining with pituitary growth hormone to increase the growth rate from a prepubertal value of about 4 cm/year to 8–10 cm/year. The growth rate then decreases until growth is complete. The endocrine influences of pubertal growth are sex steroids, growth hormone and possibly insulin, all of which increase during puberty. Pubertal growth, together with general body maturation is significantly delayed in chronic paediatric illness such as Crohn's disease or cystic fibrosis. This may cause psychological disturbance as may simple or constitutional growth delay. The most appropriate therapy for growth delay is androgens in the form of testosterone or HCG injections.

KEY WORDS: Adolescent growth spurt, sex steroids, growth delay, androgen therapy

INTRODUCTION

Growth at puberty is an important component of the process of normal linear growth. Any influence which suppresses growth during adolescence will compromise final adult height. In this chapter I will describe the auxology of pubertal growth, the hormonal interactions and influences which result in pubertal growth and finally the investigation and treatment of the common and important clinical entity of constitutional delay of growth and puberty.

AUXOLOGY

Height velocity gradually diminishes during childhood reaching levels in the region of 4 cm per year at the onset of puberty. Pubertal development is then associated with a rapid increase in height velocity

known as the adolescent growth spurt (AGS). The amplitude of the
AGS is greater in boys, where peak height velocity may reach 10.5 cm
per year compared with girls where peak height velocity averages 9.0 cm
per year. This factor in addition to the fact that pubertal growth occurs
two years later in boys, i.e. boys have two more years of prepubertal
growth (Figure 1), contribute to the difference in final adult height of
12.6 cm (5 inches) between males and females (Figure 2).

The timing of the adolescent growth spurt within puberty is of major
clinical importance. The events of puberty in boys and girls are shown
in Figures 3(a) and (b). In girls the adolescent growth spurt starts with

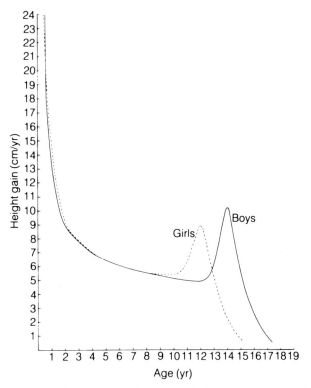

FIGURE 1   Height velocity curves in boys and girls. Note the greater amplitude and
later onset of the adolescent growth spurt in boys.

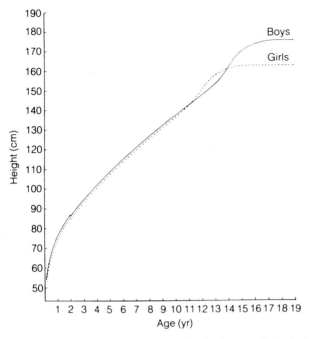

FIGURE 2   Height curves in boys and girls showing the difference in final adult height of 12.6 cm.

the onset of secondary sexual development and peak height velocity is reached at an average age of 12 years coinciding with breast development stage 4 and pubic hair stage 3. When menarche occurs, growth is already significantly decelerating. In boys, however, the onset of pubertal growth does not occur until there is significant secondary sexual development. The start of the growth spurt coincides with a testicular volume of 10 ml, measured by an orchidometer, and pubic hair stage 3. Peak height velocity occurs on average at a chronological age of 14 years coinciding with stage 4 of pubic hair development.

It is particularly important, when counselling patients with delayed growth and puberty to understand the chronology of pubertal growth. In this way it can be explained, particularly to boys, that a wait of several months may be necessary before spontaneous pubertal growth

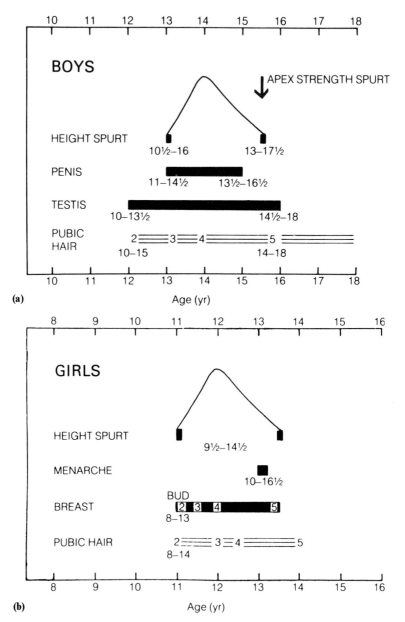

FIGURE 3   Events at puberty in boys Figure 3(a), and girls Figure 3(b). Note that the adolescent growth spurt in boys starts only at pubic hair stage 3 and testicular volume of approximately 10 ml.

occurs. Of course, there is enormous variability of the timing of puberty and of the AGS. The amplitude of the AGS is greater in early maturers than in late maturers. Late maturers may however have a greater final adult height as they have a longer period of prepubertal linear growth. The study of body proportions shows that the AGS is largely spinal in nature. Consequently in patients with delayed adolescent growth the legs continue to grow during the prepubertal period and sitting height remains more compromised. The later the AGS the more this degree of disproportion exists and patients with severe delay of puberty will ultimately have body proportions characterized by long legs and a relatively short trunk.

ENDOCRINOLOGY

A combination of hormonal influences are necessary for normal pubertal growth. Two major influences are from sex steroids, secreted during secondary sexual development, and growth hormone. A third factor which is gaining further recognition is the contribution of insulin to pubertal growth. It is well known that both the testosterone and oestradiol increase rapidly during puberty, following activation of the pituitary gonadal axis. These hormones are however not able to induce pubertal growth independently. For example, testosterone on its own will not induce a normal AGS and is dependent on a synergistic effect of growth hormone. Patterns of growth hormone pulsatility during puberty show a significant increase in primarily growth hormone pulse amplitude but also pulse frequency at the time of AGS. In patients with untreated growth hormone deficiency, the AGS will therefore be compromised. The effect of oestrogen secretion on pubertal growth has been demonstrated in patients with androgen insensitivity who have a normal AGS following a female pattern.

We know that androgens are converted by the enzyme aromatase to oestrogens in the hypothalamus and this enhancing effect of sex steroids on growth hormone may therefore occur at a hypothalamic level. This is demonstrated by the increase in peak growth hormone response to insulin-induced hypoglycaemia which occurs after stilb-oestrol-priming (Figure 4).

Fasting and stimulated concentrations of plasma insulin have

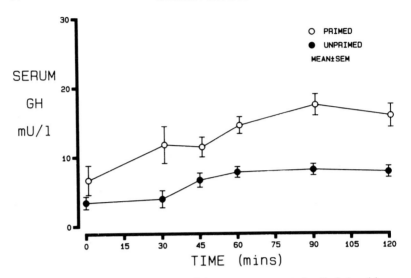

FIGURE 4   Enhancement of the growth hormone response to insulin-induced hypo-glycaemia after stilboesterol priming.

recently been shown to increase during puberty (Figure 5). Insulin concentrations similarly decline after pubertal development and linear growth is complete. The exact relationship between insulin secretion and control of height velocity during puberty has yet to be established. However it is likely that insulin contributes to this process. In summary, growth acceleration at puberty appears to be induced by a critical circulating concentration of sex steroids associated with an increase in amplitude of pulsatile growth hormone secretion. Interaction with plasma insulin may play an important contributory role.

PUBERTAL GROWTH IN CHRONIC PAEDIATRIC DISEASE

Delay of growth in childhood including pubertal growth occurs in any chronic childhood illness. Important examples are cystic fibrosis, coeliac disease, asthma and Crohn's disease. In the management of these conditions it is vital that remission should be induced if possible before the onset of pubertal growth. If puberty occurs when the patient is in a state of relapse then adolescent growth will be seriously compromised.

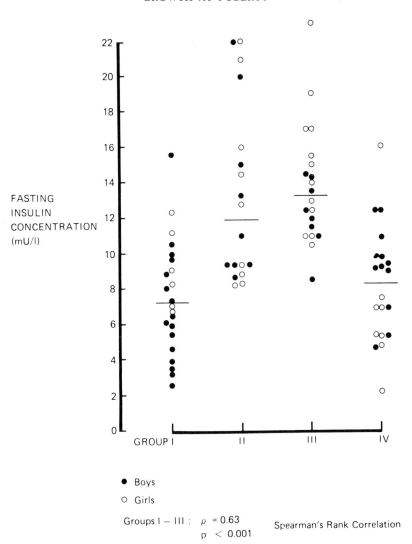

FIGURE 5   Increase in basal insulin levels during puberty in normal subjects. The patients are divided into groups (i) to (iv) according to pubertal stage. Group (i) (prepubertal subjects), group (ii) (stages 2 and 3), group (iii) (stages 3 and 4), group (iv) (normal adults). Note the increase in insulin levels during puberty followed by a decline to prepubertal levels in adult subjects.

-E

Name... Date of Birth.................... Reg. No. ....

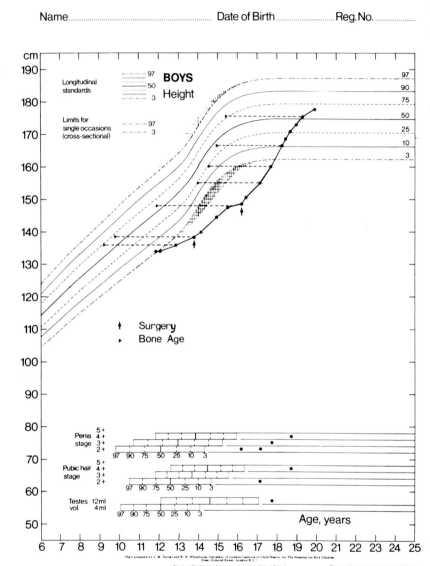

FIGURE 6   Height curve on a boy with Crohn's disease showing marked growth delay with delayed skeletal maturation, followed by catch-up growth due to remission after a second surgical procedure to remove affected bowel.

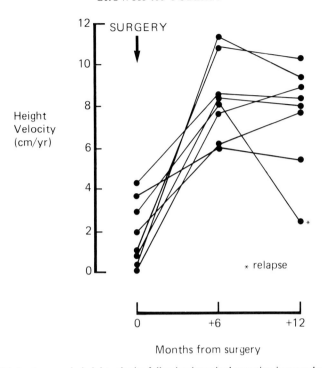

FIGURE 7   Increase in height velocity following intestinal resection in prepubertal and early pubertal subjects with Crohn's disease.

An example of the growth-depressing effect of chronic illness is seen in children with Crohn's disease. The growth chart of such a patient is shown in Figure 6. The effect of intestinal resection, i.e. removal of bowel affected by the inflammatory process of Crohn's disease, on linear growth is shown in Figure 7. When intestinal resection was performed in prepubertal or early pubertal subjects, significant catch-up growth occurred and normal of supra-normal height velocity was maintained enabling a normal AGS to occur. If surgical treatment of Crohn's disease is delayed however until a point in the process of maturation where the AGS is passed, no catch-up growth and no spontaneous pubertal growth spurt will occur.

TREATMENT OF DELAYED GROWTH AND PUBERTY

Constitutional delay of growth and puberty is the cause of significant
distress, particularly in boys. This condition is almost certainly of
heterogeneous aetiology; however the features are delayed physical
maturation associated with delayed skeletal maturation, short stature,

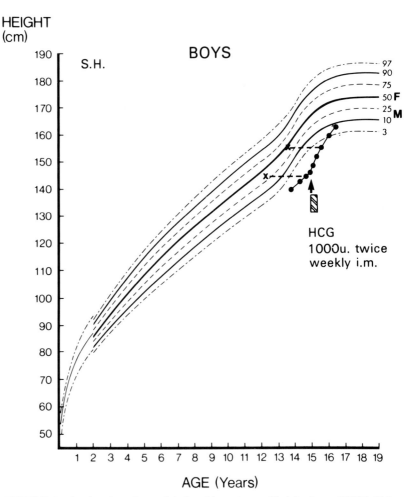

FIGURE 8   Acceleration of growth induced by twice weekly injections of HCG. This
is a physiological approach to the management of delayed growth and puberty.

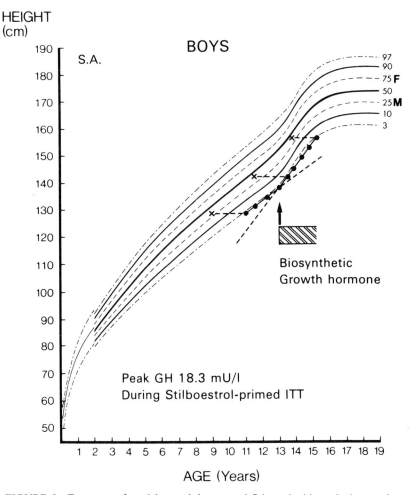

FIGURE 9 Treatment of partial growth hormone deficiency by biosynthetic growth hormone. Note that growth hormone treatment has induced a change in the axis of the height curve preventing growth delay at puberty and accompanying phychological stress.

low height velocity and delay of adolescent growth. The management of this disorder will be considered particularly in boys. A number of therapeutic possibilities exist. These are testosterone, human chorionic gonadotrophin, oxandrolone, biosynthetic growth hormone and simple observation. Testosterone therapy will induce an acceleration of linear growth and may be given as depot testosterone injections two weekly or monthly. Studies of the pharmacodynamics of injected depot testosterone indicate that circulating concentrations of testosterone will fall to basal levels rapidly and therefore the smaller the dose the more frequent are the injections indicated.

A more physiological approach is the use of human chorionic gonadotrophin (Figure 8). This is given intramuscularly on a twice weekly basis in a dose of 1,000 units per injection. Growth acceleration will be induced, associated with pubertal changes and some degree of testicular enlargement. The testes may increase to volumes of 6–8 ml. A duration of treatment of 3–6 months should be sufficient to induce symptomatic improvement of linear growth.

Biosynthetic growth hormone, if growth hormone deficiency is demonstrated, can also induce significant growth at puberty. Our patients with growth delay and a bone age of greater than 10 years, routinely have a silboestrol-primed insulin tolerance test and if the peak growth hormone is less than 20 mμ/litre, treatment with bio-synthetic growth hormone is given. The results of such treatment can be seen in Figure 9. The oral preparation Oxandrolone given as 2.5 mg daily, can induce acceleration of growth and is particularly effective in boys with testicular enlargement of greater than r ml volume. Three months therapy will accelerate pubertal growth without significant change in secondary sexual development, and may have a markedly beneficial psychological effect on the patient. The mode of action of Oxandrolone is unclear. Studies from the United States have shown that this is not accompanied by increase in pulse amplitude of growth hormone secretion. As Oxandrolone is not aromatized to oestrogen, it may have a direct growth stimulating effect independent of growth hormone secretion.

CONCLUSIONS

Growth at puberty is essential for achievement of full adult height. Deficiency of sex steroids and/or growth hormone and possibly insulin will compromise the character and amplitude of pubertal growth. The treatment of pubertal growth delay is important in boys who are particularly vulnerable to psychological distress as a result of this condition. Management of pubertal should aim for physiological hormone replacement.

Human Growth Hormone – Its Current Implications and Future Applications

BRIAN GENNERY and STEPHEN WISE

Lilly Research Centre Limited, Erl Wood Manor, Windlesham, Surrey GU20 6PH

Human growth hormone is now available in large quantities manufactured by recombinant DNA technology. This has enabled the utilisation of this product in areas outside growth hormone deficiency to begin. However, a review of the literature indicates that satisfactory evidence for efficacy and safety are not available for any new indications.

There needs to be a consensus developed as to what data is needed in order to allow registration of these new indications for marketing approvals.

The new European Community Directive on biotechnology products is encouraging the development of such areas, but there are some potential obstacles to industry being encouraged to invest in these areas.

INTRODUCTION

Growth hormone is a peptide hormone with 198 amino acid sequence, the structure of which has been well established. It has been used successfully in the treatment of growth hormone deficiency for many years now. The possible transmission of the causative virus of Jacob–Creuzefelt from cadaver growth hormone to patients accelerated the need for the development and introduction of biosynthetic human growth hormone. This has made available much larger quantities than have been possible ever before and opened up the opportunies for research into conditions other than growth hormone deficiency in childhood. This paper will describe the manufacture of biosynthetic human growth hormone, its potential wider applications and the regulatory environment surrounding biotechnology products.

PRODUCTION

In order to be able to manufacture any biosynthetic hormone it is necessary to insert the appropriate genetic information into an organism, culture that organism in large quantities and then extract and purify the product. The organism used in this particular case is an *E. coli* and Figure 1 illustrates the process by which a plasmid is extracted from a bacterium, new genetic information is inserted into the plasmid, which is then introduced into the same species once more.

This is the start point for manufacture. Organisms are taken from the seed stock and cultured in large fermenters. At the end of the fermentation the liquid and solid phases of the ferment are separated and the hormone extracted.

Chemical and biological tests are carried out to ensure that the hormone produced in this way is identical to that which occurs in nature.

PRINCIPLES OF CLINICAL RESEARCH

There are some broad goals of any clinical research programme and these can be defined as:

1. To establish initial safety in man.

2. To demonstrate the efficacy of the compound in the diseases or conditions where it is planned to be used.

3. To establish the safety profile of the compound in a large number of patients.

4. To delineate the role of the compound within the therapeutic armamentarium for the conditions under study.

5. To generate sufficient data to allow the regulatory authorities to grant permission for the compound to go on the market.

These principles should apply to the development of biosynthetic products as well as any other pharmaceutical product. In the case of

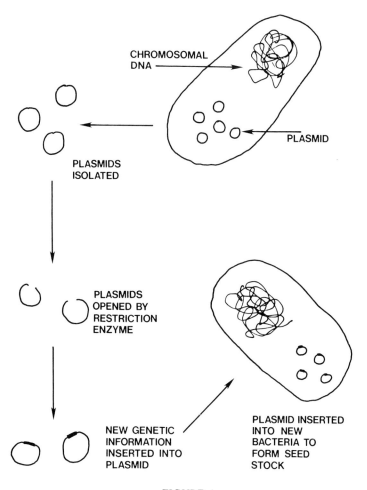

CHROMOSOMAL
DNA

PLASMID

PLASMIDS
ISOLATED

PLASMIDS
OPENED BY
RESTRICTION
ENZYME

NEW GENETIC
INFORMATION
INSERTED INTO
PLASMID

PLASMID INSERTED
INTO NEW
BACTERIA TO
FORM SEED
STOCK

FIGURE 1

biosynthetic growth hormone this has been so for the classical indication of growth hormone deficiency. It is equally important to bear these
principles in mind when considering the numerous alternative indications to which the product might be put.

FUTURE APPLICATIONS

There are a large number of potential uses for growth hormone of which three will be considered here, namely Turner's syndrome, normal variant short stature and serious wounds, especially burns.

Turner's syndrome This is a condition affecting girls where they have only one X chromosome instead of the normal 2. Recently a variant of Turner's has been described where only part of the second X chromosome is missing. The syndrome is characterised by well-known physical features. Most of the girls affected by this condition exhibit slow growth and often end up with a final height that is well below normal. However the evidence that there is a lack of growth hormone in this population is equivocal. Despite a lack of consistent data to indicate a lack of growth hormone several investigators have tried adding the hormone to the treatment of these patients.

Butenandt reported a study in which he described a total of five patients. One girl who had a GH <2 ng/ml increased her growth rate from 2 cm/yr to 4.1 cm/yr when given 10 units per metre squared per week of pituitary extracted growth hormone for one year. The four other patients who had GH levels of between 5.6 and 41 ng/ml (from below the commonly accepted lower limit of normal to well into the normal range) failed to exhibit any increase in growth rate when given up to 36 units per metre squared for the same period.

More recently Takano and associates have reported a more extensive study using biosynthetic methionyl-growth hormone. Twenty girls aged 8.4 to 16.1 years were observed for six months and then given the hormone for a further six months in a dose of 16 units per week. Sixteen of the twenty responded and their growth rate changes are given in Table I.

These early data indicate that GH may have a role to play in the

TABLE I
Growth rates

Pre-treatment	3.7 + 0.8 cm/yr
At 6 months	2.9 + 0.8 cm/yr
At 12 months	5.7 + 1.6 cm/yr

treatment of this condition and other studies are currently under way that may clarify the situation.

However, from the point of view of a pharmaceutical clinical research development programme there are still a number of unresolved questions. Some of these are:

The studies so far are small and uncontrolled.
The data is not long term.

It is unclear as to what data regulatory authorities are going to require before approving biosynthetic growth hormone for the treatment of Turner's syndrome.

Children with Normal Variant Short Stature (NVSS)   As can be seen from other contributions to this publication the very existence of this condition is open to a certain amount of debate. For many years however children who have had a growth hormone level of more than 15 ng/ml on at least one of the standard stimulation tests have been considered as not having growth hormone deficiency. Nontheless there are many children who fall below the 3rd percentile who produce much more than 15 ng/ml. The explanations as to why they do not grow as predicted are numerous and include the idea that they have resistance to growth hormone at the receptor level or that their growth hormone is of an abnormal structure and is therefore inactive.

Even before analysing what data is available it is worth setting out a number of questions for treating this condition:

Which, if any, children will show a growth spurt when given exogenous growth hormone?
Will the growth spurt be sustained?
Will treatment produce a taller or better adjusted child?
Will any adverse effects be seen?

With these questions in mind some studies have been carried out. Gertner *et al.* reported a study on ten patients. They were 9 males and 1 female aged 4.9 to 10.8 years. They all had normal levels of growth hormone on one standard stimulation test and were treated with 0.1 units per kilogramme three times a week for 6 months. Their response is shown in Table II.

This study clearly shows that a growth spurt can be induced with

TABLE II
Growth rates

Pre-treatment	4.3 + 0.3 cm/yr
At 6 months	7.4 + 0.5 cm/yr*
6 months off treatment	3.7 + 0.6 cm/yr

$* P < 0.001$ compared to pre-treatment.

TABLE III
Growth rate

Pre-treatment	3.6 + 1.6 cm/yr
At 4 months	8.6 + 4.5 cm/yr
At 8 months	7.4 + 2.9 cm/yr
At 12 months	6.8 + 2.2 cm/yr

treatment with growth hormone, but as soon as treatment is stopped then the benefit is lost immediately.

In a somewhat larger study Plotnick *et al.* treated 16 patients between the ages of 2.9 and 17.2 years at a dose of between 0.07 and 0.18 units per kilogramme 3 times a week for eight months. These results are shown in Table III.

Several points are interesting about this study. First of all not all patients responded despite the fact that the dose given differed widely. Secondly response did not correlate with acute changes in somatomedin C levels, so this was no help as guide as to whether it was worth continuing treatment or not. Finally it is interesting to note the change that occurred during the last four months of the study when the children were off treatment and their growth rate began to fall back towards pre-treatment levels.

More recently Hindmarsh and Brook have published a study on 26 children with a mean age of 8.4 years who they observed for one year. 16 of the group were then given biosynthetic methionyl–growth hormone for one year and the remaining 10 acted as controls. In the treated group growth rate increased from a pre-treatment level of 5.3 cm/yr to 7.4 cm/yr, whilst in the untreated group there was no such change. Other than the production of antibodies to the growth hormone in some of these children no adverse experiences were noted. This is also the case with the other published studies.

Thus it has been established that it is possible to make children who come into this diagnostic category to grow when given growth hormone. There are however a number of outstanding issues that need to be addressed over the coming years. They are:

1. Does the benefit in terms of growth velocity seen in the short term studies so far result in improved final height?

2. We cannot predict which children will benefit.

3. There are no data on any possible long term side effects when we expose children without demonstrable growth hormone deficiency to exogenous growth hormone.

4. Is it ethical to expose more children than are required by the scientific and statistical needs of these studies until these questions are answered?

5. No regulatory authority has yet indicated what data will be required before giving marketing approval for this indication.

These and other possible questions need to be debated and thought through before the widespread use of growth hormone can be recommended in this situation.

Possible metabolic uses of growth hormone

This is perhaps one of the most interesting, but as yet largely unexplored areas, that might exist for the use of growth hormone. The hypothesis that needs to be tested is whether growth hormone can:

1. Reverse the catabolic phase in the immediate post surgical/operative situation.

2. Improve nutrition in debilitated patients.

3. Improve the healing of wounds

A severe burn represents one of the most extreme forms of general metabolic derangement. This situation is characterised by an increase in the metabolic rate, protein catabolism, lipolysis, accelerated gluconeogenesis, muscle proteinolysis and a loss of lean body mass. Growth hormone is not the only factor involved in this problem as can be seen in Figure 2. Growth hormone levels are actually little changed after

CAUSE OF METABOLIC MANIFESTATIONS

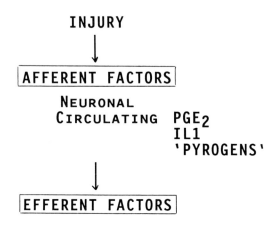

INJURY

AFFERENT FACTORS

NEURONAL
CIRCULATING   PGE$_2$
IL1
'PYROGENS'

EFFERENT FACTORS

EXCESS COUNTEREGULATORY HORMONES

FIGURE 2

burn-type injuries and may in fact be elevated. However somatomedin levels are depressed.

The therapeutic problem then is to reverse the catabolism whilst at the same time maximising the anabolism. It is important to recognise that this latter effect is only going to be possible if there is adequate food substrate available.

As early as 1956 Prudden and co-workers reported on four severely burned patients and demonstrated that compared to a control period, the nitrogen balance improved when these individuals were given growth hormone. These results have been repeated subsequently by Liljedahl et al., Soroff et al., and Wilmore et al. These data are obviously encouraging and do suggest that further studies are legitimate. As with the other potential uses of growth hormone there are a number of questions that can be set down and need to be answered before one can come to any reasonable judgement about its utility in such patients.

1. Are the changes seen in nitrogen balance translated into either shortened hospitalisation or increased survival? Carefully con-

trolled studies against placebo now need to be done to address these questions.

2. What is the optimal dose to use in these patients?

3. How long should treatment with growth hormone continue?

4. What possible side effects can be anticipated and what effect will they have on the risk/benefit ratio of this treatment?

It is clear that we are only at the beginning of the investigation of this complex area and it will be some considerable time before we can answer these questions.

THE REGULATORY CONTROL OF BIOTECHNOLOGY PRODUCTS

This is a rapidly changing area of activity which could have a significant impact on the research and development of biotechnology products in the future. All medicines are regulated in the United Kingdom by the appropriate Ministers of Health, acting on the advice of the Committee on Safety of Medicines and the Medicines Commission. We now, however, have a European dimension with regard to biotechnology products.

Under the terms of a Directive issued by the European Commission, none of the twelve member states of the European Community can authorise the marketing of a product made by a biotechnology process until the application has been reviewed by a committee in Brussels known as the Committee for Propriety Medical Products (CPMP). The actual process is illustrated in Figure 3 and, as can be seen, has imposed upon it a very strict timetable. When permission is given to market a product through this process there is then a period of 10 years in which the applicant has protection from a generic manufacturer being able to refer to the data submitted to support the original application. This is intended to stimulate investment in biotechnology in Europe by offering innovative companies protection from generic competition for a defined period of time. There is also the possibility of extensions to the original indication for the product being protected for a period of up to 6 years, although this point needs further clarification. This particular clause within the Directive is of great

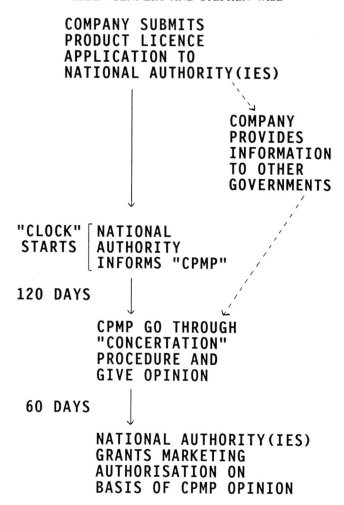

FIGURE 3

significance when looking to the future of growth hormone. The investment needed to produce enough clinical data on the various new indications is very substantial and unless there is the prospect of some protection of that data in a regulatory sense, then companies may be reluctant to commit themselves fully. This would have the exact opposite effect to what was intended by Directive.

How this develops over the next few years depends on the approach of both the various European Governments and the Commission.

CONCLUSIONS

1. Human growth hormone can be produced in a highly purified state by biotechnology in quantities to satisfy all needs.

2. The principles that govern the clinical research programme for biosynthetic human growth hormone should be the same as those that apply to any new medicinal product.

3. There is preliminary evidence that growth hormone may be useful in a variety of conditions such as Turner's syndrome, Normal Variant Short Stature and patients with severe burns.

4. There needs to be a consensus between academia, regulatory authorities and industry as to what data are going to be needed to substantiate these claims.

5. The current regulatory climate, whilst encouraging, needs to be developed to continue to stimulate research in this area.

Growth Hormone – A Consumer's Viewpoint

TAM FRY

Child Growth Foundation, 2 Mayfield Avenue, Chiswick, London W4 1PW

The author supports endocrine specialists but has little time for Health Authorities concerned with growth. He states that not every child who would benefit from growth hormone treatment will get it until the DHSS changes attitudes. Training in growth assessment and arrangements for its surveillance are woefully inadequate and the provision of growth hormone treatment wastes both resources and money.

KEY WORDS: Listen, parent, consumer, lobby, distribution, regulation, cost, surveillance, training, DHSS, Carnet, record, abuse, funding, disorders, dwarf

This chapter will aim to emphasise some of the points already made in this book but also challenge some at the same time. From the outset, and as a consumer, I must stress that the specialists who deal with hypostaturism have our complete confidence. I am afraid that other people may have less. We have a fairly low opinion of those doctors who add to the problems of families of children with growth disorders rather than helping them: of the regulatory body, of which we have heard quite often today, we have little good to say.

However, let me state first – to put this chapter in context – who I really am. I am the father of Sarah and I will tell you about Sarah because I think it will help you to understand how important height is, and how important it is to assess non-growth as early as possible. In fact, if there is one single message that I would like to leave with you, it would be "listen to the consumer – listen to the parent". At the age of three-and-a-half Sarah displayed all the symptoms, we are told, of growth hormone deficiency. It was four years later, however, that we finally managed to get a medical practitioner to listen to our concerns. Four years during which she was overtaken by her younger sister who was 18 months younger. As she grew past Sarah to an eventual seven inches taller, nobody really stopped to listen to our concerns. The story was always "she will be a late developer", "growth comes in seven year cycles". This, I am sorry to tell you, is a disgrace.

When finally she was diagnosed at the age of seven she was given a projected adult height of between 3 ft 10 ins and 4 ft. After eight years of treatment at London's Institute of Child Health she achieved the fantastic height of 5 ft $1\frac{3}{4}$ ins – the $\frac{3}{4}$ in is very important. When she was seven she was a frail, timid, introverted, shy, non-communicative person; she was so small that her size had a bearing on the family unit. My wife was very concerned; she had the feeling that it was to do with her that Sarah was the way she was. I would have found it very difficult, without Sarah's treatment, to be the father of a girl who was so out of kilter with her family background and her siblings. The fact that she has now grown has reconstituted our family into the unit that we are now. You could have seen the difference between a broken marriage and a marriage which succeeds. That is why you should bother.

One of the things we did in 1977 at the request of Professor Tanner, who was then the Professor at the Institute of Child Health, was to start a Foundation in order that other people should not have to go through the same kind of four-year trauma that we went through. I think that Professor Tanner might rue the day that he asked me to take it on since it became quite quickly apparent that what he had asked me to do was form the nucleus of a parent consumer group. Without too much problem, it would find some of the gaping holes of knowledge about growth both amongst the public in general but the medical profession in particular. And from that beginning, when we were delighted to have a £10 cheque as our first contribution to our independent charity, we have now grown into a body which not only fund raises but tries to fill those gaps.

We have been operating for ten years now, and in our eleventh year it looks as if we are going to be a lobby group as well. For there are a number of issues which must be resolved before we are likely to be satisfied that all is well with hypopituitarism. I am indebted to Dr Gennery to alluding to some of those difficulties, particularly those which encompass growth hormone, its regulation, cost and distribution. Our Foundation should not, of course, be necessary. All that we do should be done by the regulatory body whose initials I have not heard today but I will be bold enough to pronounce as DHSS. I think that the DHSS is the butt of our anger because we find it to be fairly negligent in terms of growth.

When biosynthetic growth hormone came onto the market, the Minister responsible for it, Ray Whitney, assured us that "the drug will be available to any child who would benefit from it". Although he was subsequently sacked along with his senior, we read that as a statement of government policy. But it will not materialise until a number of matters have been sorted out.

The first thing that needs to be implemented is a proper growth surveillance system for children in this country. I mean for every child, and not just for those whom you are concerned about, because it is the children whom you are not concerned about who are, in a sense, just as much at risk. The child on the 25th centile is, by all the norms, healthy; but that child is not healthy if the father and the mother are on the 97th. There is quite possibly something wrong. So I would press that every child be regularly screened in this country.

Ten years ago we were told that children were referred at an unacceptably late age for medical treatment. I think that still remains the case today but, hopefully, it will not continue too far into the future. What we would like to see is growth measurement begun at birth and continued until maturity. I know that this may raise some hackles amongst members of the audience, but that is what we believe should happen. In fact we had a study done when we first started doing seminars for the medical profession. A doctor in Wigan, disbelieving that this degree of surveillance was even possible, looked at her area with an eye to proving it. Yet she found that all that needed to be done was to add one administrative official to plot the data which was sent back by the health visitors and school nurses. She recognised that there were difficulties in measuring as well as plotting. What she envisaged was the medical profession recording the measurements, and a clerk filling out the centile charts.

We would also like to see the incredible love affair with weighing downgraded somewhat. We find that so much money is spend on sets of scales around this country, yet it is money thrown away. Charles Brook, one of my mentors in the growth business would, for one, like to dispense with scales and rely on skin fold calipers for health surveillance. He argues that skin fold measurements can tell you far more about the well being of a child than its weight.

We would like to see proper training in growth. When we ask Health Authorities if we can mount seminars in their areas we are told that they have no money, that they will not give study leave to the people to attend, that the people who wish to attend have to do it in their own leave time and, furthermore, pay their own expenses. This is unbelievably stupid. In the BBC, no engineer is allowed to work on a transmitted programme until he has undergone six months of training to tell him what the equipment is that he is using, how it is maintained and how much it costs. Yet it seems to me that a lot of nurses, school nurses, health visitors and even hospital nurses are not even taught the most fundamental things, such as how to measure. Neither are they taught what the consequences of not measuring might be. Therefore I would like to see proper training implemented in this country for those people whom we pay to look after our children's health. I am told that growth may be the best indicator of a child's well being and am disturbed that a lot of doctors, and even paediatricians, do not fully appreciate the fact.

"Biosynthetic growth hormone will be available to any child who would benefit from it" – but that will not happen until there is a national child health surveillance policy. We hold our Foundation seminars all over the place from Aberdeen to Exeter and the differences in approach from Authority to Authority staggers us. You can live in Bath and get one sort of treatment and live in Bristol and get another, and yet the cities are only 13 miles apart! Whatever you might feel about the initials "HS" being a Health Service, it is certainly not a National one. We feel that the DHSS in this respect should not be leaving it to the whim of the Regions either to concentrate on growth or not. The DHSS should be insisting that they concentrate on proper child health surveillance.

I was delighted to find that John Buckler mentions the "Carnet de santé" in his chapter. For those of you who do not know it, it is a book given to every French family on the birth of a new child which has to be completed if the parents wish to claim child benefit. I think that such a book should exist in this country. When I travel in France as a television producer I make a point of talking to my French crews about the Carnet and they cannot understand what happens in this country. They say that completing the Carnet not only encourages them to look after their children and receive benefit, but it reduces consultation time with the doctor dramatically. They find that, since all the history of their child is written down in front of them, they understand more clearly what is going on and they value very much the idea that the Carnet is retained by the parent. For those who think that parents are not responsible and cannot hold a document such as a child health record let me remind them that the same parents will unerringly hold onto their child benefit book which is smaller still. It is the greed inherent in all of us that will ensure that particular book is well looked after.

There is in the UK a commercially sponsored child health record which is hoping to do what the Carnet does. The Foundation has recommended that from now on the range of centile charts be increased from 0–2 years to 0–5 years and, I understand, this will be done from the next edition. The French Carnet contains centile charts from 0–22 years.

At a recent Foundation seminar in Birmingham, a social service team leader spoke to us about the link of growth surveillance and child abuse and, for the first time in public, I heard a welfare official admit the value of regular surveillance. He suggested that child abuse, not just sexual abuse, is noticeable as much as one year before it takes place and might be prevented if notice were taken of children's weight and height. He stressed height because emotional deprivation, as we know, can reduce height velocity and he said he has been challenging the social services to institute it. Until now, nobody has bothered but, with the events in Cleveland, he hopes that their attention has been turned to this important issue.

Now I come to the most critical point and the one which makes us particularly angry. That is that every child who may benefit from growth hormone will not receive it until the distribution and costing of the hormone is sorted out. We were told by Ray Whitney when biosynthetic growth hormone came on the market that there would be no growth, to coin a phrase, in growth hormone as a result of biosynthetic material coming into this country. Yet there is a contributor in this book whose clinic treatment list has risen 100% in the last year. For the Minister to blithely say that the introduction of recombinant growth hormone "will not increase the number of children being treated" is ridiculous.

The current system for the drug's prescription is, in our view, criminal. We can now literally run biosynthetic growth hormone out of a tap yet there are children in Wales who are being denied it. They are being denied it because of a confused situation whereby the local hospital refuses to pay for it under its pharmacy budget and their GPs refuse to prescribe it under their budgets. One-half of the DHSS creates the climate in which GPs can prescribe a very expensive drug, yet the other half says "no, you shall not prescribe". It was Len Peach, acting Chairman of the DHSS, who created this confusion. Having discovered that this £5,000 per annum hormone was being prescribed by GPs on the request of hospital consultants – the original intention – Len Peach wrote a letter to the Authorities forbidding GPs to prescribe any drug that in his view should be supplied from the hospitals where those consultants worked!

It is not for me – a mere consumer – to prescribe the solution; what I have to do is to try to ensure that every child who would benefit from hormone treatment will receive it, and it is for the civil servants in the Elephant and Castle to work out the best system to achieve that. However, a very simple solution would be some kind of central funding. This should also prevent medical abuses taking place, since some growth specialists know of GPs and paediatricians who, given the right by the DHSS to prescribe growth hormone, do not appear to know what they are doing with it. The excellence that resides in the regional centres and specialist hospitals is not some mafia clique from which the nation must be protected. It reflects the effects of a group of doctors who have concentrated on a very particular aspect of medical science and who do know what they are doing. For the DHSS to ignore their advice when they asked to retain control of growth hormone distribution, simply because it was deemed politically suitable at the time, was foolhardy. The Ministry should now think hard in favour of re-regulation if for no better reason than the bulk-buying potential which could save the NHS 40% of the purchase price of the drug. The Foundation's solution would therefore be for the DHSS to revert to the old system with central funding. The wastage caused by growth hormone distribution in this country currently runs to £1 300 000 per annum. That sum would pay for a Carnet for every baby born in this country. We could be funding a proper health record system with money that is purchasing nothing.

Of course, central funding in the present climate may simply tie the clinician's hands and prevent rather than help him treat all those who need growth hormone. Future funding has to be based on a budgeted prediction rather than on a static finite sum.

It is in this area that we, as a Foundation, would like to switch attention to the specialists themselves and ask them to form a lobby to change the present distribution system. They have not had a "lobby" since the demise of the Human Growth Hormone Committee and, unless they regroup, I fear that nothing will be done to influence current waste and abuse. Although we would recognise that the duty of the specialist is to treat children rather than be fundraisers or politicians, there is today, I am afraid, little effective alternative to the lobby.

When those three broad conditions are met, I believe every child who would benefit from growth hormone will receive it. I will not die happy until I am sure that they do. I am not talking only of hypostaturism, although growth hormone deficiency was the reason that Foundation began. I am including any disorder which may benefit from growth hormone; from Russell Silver to Turner's syndrome, hypochondroplasia to burns. The wider the benefit of growth hormone, the greater the likelihood that its price will ultimately fall. I hope that in ten years time we will no longer be talking of treatment which costs £5,000 per child per annum, but of one which the nation could more easily afford. Charles Brook once said that if you fail to give somebody the stature that they would like or deserve, the net deficit to the nation can be quantified. There was a recent programme on television about an achondroplastic who became a circus dwarf. He had not wanted to, but it was the only option open to him. He wanted to become a policeman but could not because of his size. Then he had wanted to be a fireman but could not because of his size. His next choice was the army, but he was excluded because of his size. Had he been able to achieve any of those ambitions the net benefit to the nation from a working person fulfilling his potential, would have paid for the treatment in the first place. I believe that the nation can ill afford not to treat small people wherever they may benefit.

INDEX